MEDIC D1764945

Chronic Mental Illness

Series Editor
John A. Talbott, University of Maryland School of Medicine,
Baltimore, USA

Advisory Board
Leona Bachrach • James T. Barter • Carol Caton • David L. Cutler
• Jeffrey L. Geller • William M. Glazer • Stephen M. Goldfinger •
Howard H. Goldman • H. Richard Lamb • Harriet P. Lefley •
Anthony F. Lehman • Robert P. Lieberman • W. Walter Menninger
• Arthur T. Meyerson

Mentally Ill and Homeless

Special Programs for Special Needs

Edited by

William R. Breakey, MB, FRCPsych

The Johns Hopkins University School of Medicine
Baltimore, Maryland

and

James W. Thompson, MD, MPH

University of Maryland School of Medicine
Baltimore, Maryland

harwood academic publishers

Australia Canada China France Germany India
Japan Luxembourg Malaysia The Netherlands Russia
Singapore Switzerland Thailand

Amsteldijk 166
1st Floor
1079 LH Amsterdam
The Netherlands

British Library Cataloguing in Publication Data

Mentally ill and homeless : special programs for special
    needs. − (Chronic mental illness ; v. 6)
    1. Mentally ill − Housing − United States   2. Homeless persons
    − Mental health − United States   3. Housing policy − United
    States
    I. Breakey, William R.   II. Thompson, James W.
    362.2′086942′0973

    ISBN 90-5702-557-4

CONTENTS

INTRODUCTION TO THE SERIES

This series on chronic mental illness is a result of both the success and failure of our efforts over the past thirty years to provide better treatment, rehabilitation and care for persons suffering from severe and persistent mental illnesses. The failure is obvious to all who walk our cities' streets, use our libraries or pass through our transportation terminals. The success is found in the enormous boost of interest in service to, research on and teaching about treatment, rehabilitation and care of those persons who, in Leona Bachrach's definition, "are, have been, or might have been, but for the deinstitutionalization movement, on the rolls of long-term mental institutions, especially state hospitals."

The first book in our modern era devoted to the subject was that by Richard Lamb in 1976, *Community Survival for Long-Term Patients.* Shortly thereafter, Leona Bachrach's unique study "Deinstitutionalization: An Analytical Review and Sociological Perspective" was published. In 1978, the American Psychiatric Association hosted a meeting on the problem that resulted in the publication *The Chronic Mental Patient.* This effort in turn spawned several texts dealing with increasingly specialized areas: *The Chronic Mentally Ill: Treatment, Programs, Systems* and *Chronic Mental Illness in Children and Adolescents,* both by John Looney; and *The Chronic Mental Patient/II* by Walter Menninger and Gerald Hannah.

Now, however, there are a host of publications devoted to various portions of the problem, e.g., the homeless mentally ill, rehabilitation of the mentally ill, families of the mentally ill and so on. The amount of research and experience now that can be conveyed to a wide population of caregivers is exponentially greater than it was in 1955, the year that deinstitutionalization began.

This series will cover:

— types of intervention, e.g., psychopharmacology, psychotherapy, case management, social and vocational rehabilitation and mobile and home treatment;
— settings, e.g., hospitals, ambulatory settings, nursing homes, correctional facilities and shelters;
— specific populations, e.g., alcohol and drug abusers, the homeless and those dually diagnosed;

— special issues, e.g., family intervention, psychoeducation, policy/
  financing, non-compliance, forensic, cross-cultural and systems
  issues.

I am indebted to our hard-working editorial board as well as to our
editors and authors, many of whom are involved in both activities.

   This sixth volume deals with the subject that so many of us in the
field have struggled with ever since the excesses of deinstitutionalization reached public and professional awareness — the homeless
mentally ill. Its editors are both skilled and experienced academic and
practical psychiatrists, well known for their high quality research and
service. The book's contributors are equally able to address the many
complex facets of this population that occupy us to this day.

   Future books in the series will deal with the issues of sexuality,
inpatient care, ethics and psychopharmacology — all as related to
the treatment, care and rehabilitation of the chronic mentally ill. I
hope you'll look forward to them as much as I do.

John A. Talbott, MD

PREFACE

The fact that some mentally ill Americans are homeless and living on the streets has, since the early 1980s, outraged the public and been a visible sign of the failures of some of our social and health care policies. The homelessness of many people with disabling mental illnesses has led psychiatrists and mental health service researchers and providers to seek methods and strategies to understand the phenomenon of homelessness and to develop ways to address the needs of homeless individuals with severe mental illnesses.

The extent of mental pathology among homeless people has been well documented and its particular relationship to mental illness explored. Two main issues confront us: How can we prevent mentally disabled people from falling through the gaps in our service systems and ending up on the streets? How can we best address the needs of homeless mentally ill people? This book is mainly concerned with the second question — meeting the mental health service needs of people with disabling mental illnesses who are homeless.

Models have been developed for outreach, mobile service provision, shelter-based clinics and other approaches, and most large cities can now boast one or more programs offering front-line mental health care to homeless people. Problems persist, however, with reintegrating homeless or formerly homeless mentally ill people into the mainstream of society and into the mainstream mental health service system. Enormous challenges are presented in coordinating the complex set of services needed by people who are homeless and mentally disabled, and helping them gain entitlements, get access to suitable housing arrangements, settle into new surroundings and handle new responsibilities.

As part of its contribution to the effort, the National Institute of Mental Health, implementing provisions of the McKinney Homelessness Act, funded a series of research-demonstration projects in 1990 to develop and evaluate novel approaches to meeting the needs of people who are homeless and mentally ill. Six projects got under way: one in each of four cities — Baltimore, Boston, Cincinnati, San Diego — and two in New York. These projects addressed specific needs: outreach to the streets where homeless people are to be found; transitional services to sustain them during transition from shelter living to the community; supportive housing programs to enable them to resettle in more normal environments; rehabilitation services to help them develop needed skills; and use of case management approaches to help individuals settle permanently once they have been rehoused.

Descriptions of all six projects form the central core of this book; the authors are the researchers who undertook the six experiments. They write from personal experience gained as they struggled with the clinical, administrative, political and personal problems encountered in helping this special population. Each program has been very carefully evaluated, using state-of-the-art mental health service research methods. Detailed findings of the research will be published elsewhere; these chapters provide only hints as to outcomes, or summaries of data. The purpose of this book is, rather, to describe experiences; outline successes and failures of clinical approaches as well as research strategies; share practical insights of these pioneers; and provide guidance for others who may wish to pursue similar endeavors. Of the six programs, the one in Cincinnati failed to establish itself. Experiences of that research team are included here so that others might learn from them.

Because the work of the McKinney researchers built upon what had been learned about homelessness and mental illness over the period of a decade, an introductory chapter reviews the state of our knowledge before the six McKinney projects got under way. Much of this knowledge had been acquired by clinicians and investigators working with funding support of the National Institute of Mental Health and articulated in a series of NIMH conferences and reports. Chapter 2, authored by federal officials responsible for overseeing the McKinney projects, describes the federal role in addressing "social problems," and the process by which the federal government agency identified an issue and pursued it systematically over a decade. After each research group describes its project and what members think are the most important insights gained from the work, a final chapter presents a summing up of lessons learned from this program of research and points to some directions for the future.

This volume is written for those who work with homeless people, do research in this area, or wish to get involved. It provides many practical insights into the organization of service programs for homeless mentally ill people and the challenge of conducting empirical research in these settings.

CONTRIBUTORS

Mark S. Abelman, MSW, Senior Program Director, Bay Cove Human Services, Inc., Boston, Massachusetts.

William A. Anthony, PhD, Executive Director, Center for Psychiatric Rehabilitation, Boston University.

Tara L. AvRuskin, PhD candidate, Department of Anthropology, Harvard University.

William R. Breakey, MB, FRCPsych, Professor, Department of Psychiatry and Behavioral Sciences, The Johns Hopkins University School of Medicine.

Joshua Breslau, PhD candidate, Department of Anthropology, Harvard University.

Brina Caplan, EdD, PhD, Instructor in Psychology, Department of Psychiatry, Harvard Medical School.

Mikal Cohen, PhD, Associate Director, Center for Psychiatric Rehabilitation, Boston University.

Sarah Conover, MPH, Research Scientist, Epidemiology and Community Psychiatry, New York State Psychiatric Institute.

Nancy Cope, PhD, Counseling Psychologist, New York, New York.

Areta Crowell, PhD, Director, Los Angeles County Mental Health Services.

Bruce R. DeForge, PhD, Assistant Professor, Director of Research, Family Medicine Department, University of Maryland Medical Systems.

Barbara Dickey, PhD, Associate Professor, Department of Psychiatry, Harvard Medical School.

Lisa Dixon, MD, Associate Professor, Center for Mental Health Services Research, University of Maryland School of Medicine.

Alan Felix, MD, Assistant Clinical Professor, Department of Psychiatry, Columbia University.

Janet Ford, Assistant Professor, University of Kentucky College of Social Work.

Beverly Gentry, MSW, Former Research Associate, Hamilton County Community Mental Health Board, Cincinnati, Ohio.

Stephen M. Goldfinger, MD, Vice Chairman, Department of Psychiatry, Downstate Medical Center, State University of New York, Brooklyn, New York.

Olinda Gonzalez, PhD, Researcher/Consultant, Washington, DC.

Byron Good, PhD, Professor of Medical Anthropology, Department of Social Medicine, Harvard Medical School.

Stephen Harmon, MS, La Jolla, California.

James E. Healy, BA, Evaluation Coordinator, Hamilton County Community Mental Health Board, Cincinnati, Ohio.

Sondra J. Hellman, RNCS, Director, Continuing Care Service, Massachusetts Mental Health Center; Instructor in Administration, Harvard Medical School.

James R. Hillard, MD, Chairman, Department of Psychiatry, University of Cincinnati College of Medicine.

Richard L. Hough, PhD, Principal Investigator, Child & Family Research, San Diego State University and University of California, San Diego.

Michael Hurlburt, PhD, Research Associate, Homeless Research Project, San Diego, California.

Eimer Kernan, MSW, Project Coordinator, Center for Mental Health Services Research, University of Maryland School of Medicine.

Nancy Krauss, LCSW-C, Program Director, UMMS ACT Team, Baltimore, Maryland.

Paula Landau-Cox, LCSW, Chief, Case Management Services, San Diego County Mental Health Services.

Susan Soyoung Lee, PhD candidate, Department of Clinical Psychology, University of Massachusetts at Boston.

Anthony Lehman, MD, MSPH, Professor of Psychiatry, Director, Center for Mental Health Services Research, University of Maryland School of Medicine.

Irene S. Levine, PhD, Research Scientist, Nathan S. Kline Institute for Psychiatric Research, Orangeburg, New York.

Ron Milone, MA, Program Manager, North County Interfaith Council, Escondido, California.

Elizabeth Morris, MA, Executive Director, San Diego Housing Commission.

Robert L. Obermeyer, BA, Chief Operating Officer, Hamilton County Community Mental Health Board, Cincinnati, Ohio.

Martha O'Bryan, RN, Director of Special Projects, Comprehensive Behavioral Care, Tampa, Florida.

Fred C. Osher, MD, Director, Division of Community Psychiatry, University of Maryland Medical School.

Walter E. Penk, PhD, Chief, Psychology Service, Edith Norse Rogers Memorial Veterans Hospital, Bedford, Massachusetts.

Robert Quinlivan, LCSW, Director, Telecare Corporation, San Diego, California.

Virginia Renker, BA, Research Director, Homeless Research Project, San Diego, California.

Donald G. Rohner, BA, Former Associate Executive Director, Hamilton County Community Mental Health Board, Cincinnati, Ohio.

Russell K. Schutt, PhD, Professor and Chair of Sociology, University of Massachusetts at Boston.

Larry J. Seidman, PhD, Associate Professor of Psychology, Department of Psychiatry, Harvard Medical School.

David L. Shern, PhD, Dean and Professor, Florida Mental Health Institute, University of South Florida, Tampa.

Roger B. Straw, PhD, Chief, Review Planning and Program Coordination Branch, Office of Extramural Activities Review, Substance Abuse and Mental Health Services Administration, Rockville, Maryland.

Ezra Susser, MD, DrPH Associate Professor of Psychiatry, Columbia University.

Henry Tarke, LCSW, Central Region Manager, San Diego County Mental Health Services.

James W. Thompson, MD, MPH, Associate Professor, Department of Psychiatry, University of Maryland School of Medicine.

George Tolomiczenko, PhD, MPH, Mental Health Researcher, Clark Institute of Psychiatry, Toronto, Ontario.

Julio Torres, MDiv, Director of Training and Clinical Development, Columbia-Presbyterian Critical Time Intervention, Mental Health Program for the Homeless, New York, New York.

Sam Tsemberis, PhD, Director, Pathways to Housing, New York, New York.

Winston M. Turner, PhD, Associate in Health Policy, Department of Psychiatry, Massachusetts General Hospital, Boston.

Elie Valencia, JD, MA, Assistant Clinical Professor of Public Health (Sociomedical Sciences) in Psychiatry, College of Physicians and Surgeons, Columbia University.

Norma Ware, PhD, Assistant Professor of Medical Anthropology, Department of Social Medicine, Harvard Medical School.

Jim Winarski, MSW, Director of Training, Better Homes Fund, Newton, Massachusetts.

Patricia A. Wood, MPH, Research Associate, Homeless Research Project, San Diego, California.

Sandra Yamashiro, MPA, Principal Analyst, San Diego County Mental Health Services, California.

1

Psychiatric Services for Mentally Ill Homeless People

WILLIAM R. BREAKEY and
JAMES W. THOMPSON

The purpose of this chapter is to set the stage for what follows. For more than a decade, American psychiatrists and other mental health professionals and service providers have worked to understand homelessness as it affects people with serious mental illness. Here we outline the current state of practice in this field, to provide a context for the descriptions of innovative new programs which follow.

Psychiatric epidemiologists had demonstrated as early as the 1960s that the prevalence of psychiatric disorders was high among American homeless people, such as those who frequented the Bowery in New York (Spitzer *et al.*, 1969). It was not until the late 1970s, however, that the issue was compellingly brought to the attention of American psychiatry (Reich & Siegel, 1978) and not until the 1980s that, stimulated by the National Institute of Mental Health, significant programs of research and service development got under way (Tessler & Dennis, 1989). An issue which had been largely ignored by all but a small group of researchers over the preceding decades became a major focus of mental health epidemiology and social research in the 1980s (Fig. 1.1).

In the past decade the problem of homelessness in the United States has become more severe and there has been little overall improvement in the plight of the homeless mentally ill. After ten years of research and program development, however, the nature and extent of the problems are better documented and there has been progress in developing treatment, rehabilitation and resettlement approaches (Institute of Medicine, 1988; Burt & Cohen, 1989;

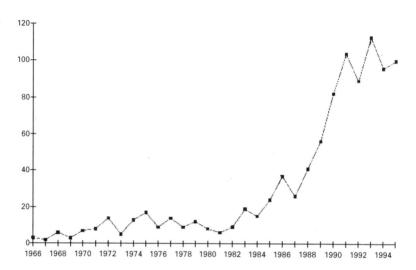

Figure 1.1. Citations of *Health* and *Homelessness* in the medical literature, 1966–1993, based on literature searches using Medline (Dellon, 1996, Personal Communication).

Jahiel, 1992; Robertson & Greenblatt, 1992; Brickner *et al.*, 1990; Lamb, Bachrach & Kass, 1992).

EXTENT OF THE PROBLEM

The first priority of research in homelessness and mental illness was to document the extent and nature of the psychiatric problems of homeless people (Fischer & Breakey, 1991). In the mid-1980s there were several prevalence studies in major American cities. They found that prevalence rates of specific psychiatric disorders vary in different subgroups of homeless people and from place to place, but a broad consensus emerged that of homeless people residing in shelters, about one third had significant mental illnesses. This estimate was derived from reports that about one third have been admitted to a psychiatric inpatient facility at some time, but documented more precisely by carefully designed surveys of homeless people using standardized diagnostic methods (Farr, Koegel & Burnam, 1986; Breakey *et al.*, 1989; Susser *et al.*, 1989; Smith, North & Spitznagel, 1992, 1993). Data from the Baltimore Homeless Study are typical (Table 1.1). Approximately 35 percent of men and 48 percent of women were found to have a major mental illness: schizophrenia was diagnosed in 9 percent of men and 16 percent of women, and major affective disorders in 17 percent of men and 25 percent of women. Note that these mentally ill people varied in their degree of disability, as do mentally ill people in general. If criteria of extensive histories of inpatient admissions and significant functional impairment are

Table 1.1. The Baltimore Homeless Study: prevalence of DSM-III psychiatric disorders (percent).

		Men	Women
MAJOR MENTAL ILLNESSES			
Schizophrenia:	total	9.0	16.3
	SM[1]	7.3	10.3
Bipolar disorder:	total	4.7	9.7
	SM[1]	1.3	9.3
Major depression:	total	12.6	13.8
	SM[1]	6.3	2.3
Other major mental illnesses[2]:	total	8.3	8.3
	SM[1]	2.0	1.8
SUBSTANCE USE DISORDERS			
Alcohol abuse or dependence		67.0	26.2
Other drug use disorder		28.8	11.1
Dual diagnosis (major mental illnesses + substance use disorder)		24.7	24.3
OTHER DSM-III AXIS I DISORDERS		30.0	46.2
PERSONALITY (DSM-III AXIS II) DISORDERS		46.5	45.3

[1]Severely mentally ill: mental illness diagnosis, with history of extensive hospitalization and/or severe functional impairment.
[2]Includes paranoid disorder, atypical psychosis, organic hallucinosis, etc.

applied to those patients with major mental illnesses, the number who are severely mentally ill is many fewer. It is this group, 17 percent of men and 24 percent of women in the Baltimore sample, who present the greatest needs for treatment and rehabilitation.

The high levels of morbidity documented in these studies are a cause, and in some cases a result of, their homelessness. First, as to how homelessness can have traumatic effects on people: poverty is stressful, the streets are dangerous and homeless people are especially prone to be victims of assault and robbery. Some people, particularly women, have become homeless as a result of unbearable or abusive relationships, while others have suffered the indignities of unemployment and eviction. Understandably, stresses such as these may produce a variety of emotional responses, exacerbate existing illnesses and increase the likelihood of substance abuse.

Second, many homeless people have become vulnerable, and thus ultimately homeless, *because* of disability produced by mental illness or dependence on alcohol or other drugs. Although psychiat-rically disabled persons are eligible for Social Security and other income supports, the level of these payments is insufficient to raise the person out of poverty, and of limited benefit to a person whose money management skills may be compromised by illness or cogni-tive impairment.

HETEROGENEITY OF THE POPULATION

Experience and research findings have led to an appreciation of the heterogeneity of homeless people. Homeless people do not consti-tute a distinct class of individuals, alienated from the mainstream of society, often threatening to, or challenging, the general population of domiciled people. The notion of an underclass has given way to a view of homelessness as a state into which people arrive for a wide variety of reasons. The homeless population thus contains a number of subgroups of poor people who end up on the streets or in the shelters who may have different profiles of disorders. For example, a survey of mothers in shelters for families in Massachusetts revealed a profile of psychiatric disorders in these young women which was different from that observed in studies of older, single homeless people. Personality disorders were more frequent and major mental illnesses less frequent (Bassuk, Rubin & Lauriat, 1986). Other studies of women have found high prevalence rates of post-traumatic stress disorder (Smith, North & Spitznagel, 1993).

POVERTY

The heterogeneity of homeless people notwithstanding, they have in common their poverty. Homeless individuals are in many respects similar to low-income housed people; indeed those who are the housed poor this week may become the homeless poor next week. The degree of instability in the residential arrangements of poor people varies considerably, so that it makes sense to think of a continuum of residential stability (Appleby & Desai, 1987; Breakey & Fischer, 1995).

The association of mental illness and poverty has been well docu-mented; the prevalence of mental illnesses, notably schizophrenia, is highest in the lowest socio-economic groups (Cohen, 1993; Holzer *et al.*, 1986). Poverty, superimposed upon their disabilities and their disaffiliation places people with severe mental illnesses at risk of homelessness. Solving the problem of homelessness will entail addressing the causes of poverty in the midst of affluence – for the mentally ill as much as for anyone else.

DISAFFILIATION

Although homeless people may develop circles of acquaintances who support one another in certain ways, in general they suffer from a lack of the networks of personal support which other people rely upon to connect them to wider circles of supportive relationships. Linkages to family, to friends, to neighbors, to churches, to occupational or other social groupings are lacking or fragmentary. In most cases they characterize themselves as loners. Disaffiliation and isolation make it more difficult for them to cope with life's hardships. In therapy with homeless patients, the lack of family and social networks deprives them of a source of support which is ordinarily available in the treatment and rehabilitation of other psychiatric patients. What is more, those personal attributes which impair a person's ability to develop and maintain social networks also impair the capacity to establish effective therapeutic relationships. Homeless people are often cautious in their relationships, frequently distrust authority and are suspicious of psychiatrists and other mental health professionals. They may have had bad experiences with hospitals or doctors which lead them to be wary of further involvement. Some former patients who have experienced unpleasant medication side-effects choose to stay away from psychiatrists to avoid being pressured into another course of treatment

RESPONDING TO THE NEED

Since the mid-1980s, agencies providing services to homeless people, community psychiatrists and other mental health care providers have struggled to develop appropriate responses to meeting the mental health service needs of homeless people, particularly the severely mentally ill. With their accumulating experiences, a number of principles have emerged.

First, mental health programs must recognize that there are several subgroups of homeless people, each of which has its own profile of needs (Fischer & Breakey, 1986). These include the *street people*, often eccentric and bizarre individuals who have made the streets their home, many of whom are chronically mentally ill; *chronic alcoholics*, whose activities center around satisfying the craving for alcohol; *situationally homeless* people, whose homelessness has resulted from a change in circumstances, such as unemployment, spousal abuse or urban redevelopment; and the *chronically mentally ill short term homeless group*, whose mental illness interferes with their capacity to settle in a stable housing arrangement and function socially, but are not socialized to street dwelling to the same extent as the Street People. Among the mentally ill, the most difficult to treat are those with comorbid substance use disorders, the *dually diagnosed*. Other subgroups with special needs are *homeless families*, now estimated to comprise perhaps 20 percent of the homeless population, *homeless children and adolescents*, living on the streets of major cities and people with *HIV infection*, many of whom are also substance abusers.

Second, homeless people, more than most, present to the service provider a multiplicity of needs. There are very few simple or uncomplicated cases. Apart from assistance with obtaining shelter, clothing, food, financial support and other basic needs, their physical health is often very poor. They not only suffer from the same disorders that affect others, but also from physical problems that are especially common because of their peculiar lifestyle. Infectious diseases, parasitic diseases, respiratory diseases, dermatological and orthopedic problems are common, in addition to the results of trauma and the complications of substance abuse (Breakey et al., 1989; Gelberg & Linn, 1989; Wright, 1990). HIV disease and AIDS are of major concern in homeless people (Susser et al., 1993).

Third, substance abuse disorders are ubiquitous (Fischer, 1990). Any treatment program for the homeless must expect that 40 to 60 percent of patients, including those whose primary diagnosis is schizophrenia or a major affective disorder, will have substance abuse or dependence and should plan accordingly. Alcohol and other drug dependence have traditionally been the major disorders of homeless people. With attention focused recently on mental illness, less public prominence has been accorded to issues of substance abuse and dependence. Again, data from Baltimore are typical of data from other American cities in showing that alcoholism and drug use are extremely prevalent, occurring in two thirds of men and one third of women.

Four Stages of Service Provision

There are four principal stages in providing psychiatric services for homeless people: engagement, basic service provision, transition, and integration.

Engagement: Gaining a person's confidence to the point where he or she will enter treatment is often a major issue because of the reluctance of many homeless mentally ill people to accept help, their fear of being forced into hospital or into accepting treatment they do not want, or their lack of insight into the fact that they are ill. It is not sufficient to establish a clinical service program and expect severely disabled homeless people to come in spontaneously for services. Thus health programs for homeless people are often located in areas where homeless people already congregate – such as shelters, skid rows, or in mobile units or temporary buildings which can be strategically placed for maximum accessibility. One of the first psychiatrists to take seriously the need for special services for the homeless was Roger Farr who established a clinical program on Skid Row in Los Angeles (Farr, 1986; Lomas, 1992). It was clear that homeless mentally ill people were not going to come to a conventional clinic, so he went to where they were. Others have confirmed that the only way to be accessible to homeless people is to take the services to those places where homeless people normally congregate. Valencia and Susser and their colleagues (Susser et al., 1993) work within a massive shelter in New York, and the health care program for homeless people in Baltimore began its operations within two daytime walk-in shelters in the city. There are many other examples. Still, it is necessary to reach out beyond the walls of the clinic or shelter. Many programs employ outreach workers who go to the streets and alleys, parks and railroad stations (Susser *et al.*, 1992). Several, such as that in Milwaukee (Blackwell, 1990) have developed multi-disciplinary outreach teams.

Outreach is an ideal staff role for formerly homeless people, whose knowledge of the territory and ability to establish rapport with homeless people is frequently superior to that of most professionals. An outreach worker or outreach team's role is, first, to establish contact with a person in need, then gain his or her confidence, which may take many contacts over a long period of time, and then to persuade the individual to accept help. Ovrebo (1992) notes that professional help is often seen as a direct path to institutionalization, which means loss of autonomy and self-respect. This perception is quite contrary to reality. Lomas (1992) notes that individuals cared for in the Los Angeles Skid Row mental health program are likely to experience less institutional care than in the period prior to their entry to the program. Diagnostic and treatment services may be brought to a person on the street, or the person may be persuaded to go to a clinic or service center, where help is available. (Figure 1.2)

Not all homeless people require long periods of persuasion and familiarization before they are willing to accept psychiatric help. Many, who have benefited from previous treatment, are grateful that services are made available to them. Whichever is the case, a range of basic services will be needed to assist the individual.

Basic Service provision: Shelter is a first requirement for those who have been living rough. Income support, clothing, and general health care will be needed in most cases, in addition to whatever psychiatric treatment may be indicated. Homeless people themselves are clear about the existence of a hierarchy of needs. Ball and Havassy (1984), for example, listed the needs expressed by homeless mentally ill people in San Francisco. Mental health treatment

---

Mental Health Services for Homeless People

ENGAGEMENT

BASIC SERVICES

TRANSITION

INTEGRATION

Figure 1.2. Mental Health Services for Homeless People

was far down the list. Herman, Struening and Barrow (1993) found in a survey of shelter users in New York, that while the interviewers considered that mental health services were needed by 41 percent of those surveyed, only 17 percent of the homeless people themselves thought that they needed mental health services. First priority in their minds went to housing, food, clothing and money. It is unrealistic to expect homeless people to participate in treatment programs until their basic needs have been met. Psychiatric treatment providers, therefore, must work closely in concert with providers of basic subsistence needs. Some services are needed to meet the special needs of homeless people. For example, a mailing address is generally necessary to receive a Social Security check. In some cases, where a person has a documented history of poor money management, a representative payee is needed. A homeless service center can provide an address, or, with the implementation of proper procedures and safeguards, act as representative payee. Purchasing medications, and storing them safely, can be a major difficulty for a person living on the street. Providing facilities for storing medicines can be an extremely helpful service (Lomas, 1992).

Coordinating the various social and health agencies can be a challenging problem. In some cases it may be facilitated by setting up multidisciplinary teams of social workers, nurses, psychiatrists and advocates; basing mental health clinics in centers which provide a number of services under one roof is helpful. Case management, however, has come to be the major strategy employed. A case manager's primary role is to ensure that the variety of services needed by a particular person are made available. The task involves evaluation of the individual's particular set of needs, coordination of the several service systems, support of the client, and advocacy, where barriers to service have to be overcome (Billig & Levinson, 1987; Goering & Wasylenki, 1996; Swayze, 1992).

Clinical services needed for homeless people cover the full range of services generally provided by a community mental health center. Diagnosis and evaluation, pharmacological and psychotherapeutic treatments and coordination with general health care providers are first provided at outpatient level. Inpatient admissions are needed in some cases, and for this, good relations with psychiatric hospitals or units are essential. Homeless patients are not only poor, but often considered to be unattractive, "problem" patients, and arranging post-hospital disposition is likely to be very difficult. Hospital admission offices may therefore try to avoid admitting homeless people. The homeless service provider must thus develop good working professional relations with the hospital staff, so that when an admission is needed, it can be arranged with a minimum of obstruction.

Transition: The third and fourth stages, transition and integration, present the greatest challenges and are a major focus of the experimental programs described in the later chapters of this book. Community mental health programs understand that their patients with severe and persistent mental illnesses in all probability will require treatment for life. On the other hand, programs for homeless people can not, by definition, provide indefinite care for people.

Once a person has been engaged, and basic service needs met, he or she must be moved into the mainstream mental health service system. This may take time. The very reason for their being in a special program for homeless people may have been their reluctance to enter the mainstream service system (Surber *et al.*, 1988). The therapist will therefore need to engage the patient, establish trust, and then use this trusting relationship to enable the transition to another treatment provider. For a while the patient will become a regular client of the homeless program. When the idea of moving the patient to another setting is broached, it is likely to be perceived by the patient as yet another in a series of rejections which may have been lifelong. For the therapist, transferring a patient with whom he or she is working effectively is also a loss, and may be consciously or unconsciously resisted. Nevertheless, mental health programs for homeless people are generally limited in their resources and unable to care for very large numbers of people. Patients can generally be helped to understand this and to accept the need to move on to a mainstream clinical setting.

Integration: In the fourth stage, the person moves out of settings and programs designed for homeless people, into the general community, with regular housing and other supports. This is an area that has been relatively little documented. To what extent can homeless people lose their identity of "homeless" or "formerly homeless", and what will facilitate this?

The success of this final step depends on the ability of the mainstream mental health service system to accept and retain patients who may be reluctant particiants. Case managers and clinicians may need to make special efforts to ensure that the formerly homeless person integrates effectively into the culture of the program and the community, recognizing that formerly homeless people are more vulnerable than others to slip back into homelessness.

The consumer movement has had considerable impact on thinking about services for homeless people in recent years, as it has in other areas of public life and in community mental health. Organizations of homeless and formerly homeless people have had important roles, through advocacy and confrontation, in sensitizing the public and those in power to the dilemmas homeless people face. Service programs increasingly incorporate consumers or former consumers into their teams. Consumer-run programs have been able to reach out to homeless people in ways that may be more effective than conventional professional approaches (Van Tosh, 1993).

CLINICAL AND PROGRAMMATIC CONSIDERATIONS

As the words "homeless mentally ill" indicate, there are two broad strategic objectives: to treat the illness and to end the homelessness. At each stage, both objectives need to be kept in mind. Without treating the illness, the person may have great difficulty in obtaining or retaining housing; without addressing the housing problem, attempts at treatment of the mental illness will be futile.

In many cases, homeless patients are among the most severely and chronically ill that a therapist is likely to encounter. They often are "treatment resistant" and have minimal resources in material terms as well as in terms of their social environment. To avoid disillusionment, it is wise to keep in mind that the prognosis in many cases is poor. Some homeless people may be reluctant to contemplate a change in their lifestyle, or may not believe that a better way of life is feasible for them. For some it seems as if the street offers a haven of anonymity, an environment to which they have made a bizarre adjustment, but one which satisfies their needs. Some have developed a routine whereby their needs are met, albeit at marginal subsistence level, and for them adjusting to a new, domiciled lifestyle would be too much to contemplate. They have achieved a level of competence in coping with a dangerous, even hostile environment, and to leave that environment for another, in which their incompetence would be all too apparent, is not an attractive prospect. So when help is offered along conventional lines, homeless people may reject it (Drake & Adler, 1984). Often a clinician must exercise great patience to establish trust. Simply offering a friendly word, or some food or clothing, may be all that is possible at first. Over time, as trust develops, more active interventions become possible.

A consideration of the many tasks and skills involved in providing services to homeless people indicates the necessity of team work. A psychiatrist, psychologist, nurse or social worker working alone can certainly be of assistance to many people, but to provide an adequate service requires the efforts of a team of specialists who combine their skills. Clinical teams that provide mental health services for homeless patients typically include psychiatrists, nurses, social workers, case managers, substance abuse specialists, patient advocates and outreach workers, some of whom are likely to be formerly homeless people.

As with the treatment of mentally ill patients anywhere in any setting, from time to time it becomes necessary to consider involuntary treatment. Because of their vulnerability to exploitation, their lifestyle and their apparent rejection of the norms of conventional living, the issue of involuntary treatment for homeless mentally ill people is particularly controversial and requires great sensitivity on the part of service providers. Opinions are divided as to whether a mentally ill person's right to independence and self-determination should be repeated even where his or her behavior is endangering his or her own health and is offensive to other citizens. The view is sometimes expressed that restrictions on involuntary admission should be relaxed so that seriously ill people can be more easily hospitalized, that this respects their right to treatment, even when they are unable to consent to it, and that admitting a person to a substandard facility is the lesser of two evils, when compared to having a person stay on the streets (Lamb, Bachrach, Goldfinger & Kass, 1992). However many of those who work in the field are of the opinion that the great majority of mentally ill people can be treated or sheltered without resorting to involuntary treatment procedures, and that, instead of looking to institutional models of care, policy makers' attention should be focused upon the great poverty of many mentally ill people, the lack of suitable housing, and the need for better community support systems which might prevent their homelessness. What is more, Appelbaum (1992) points out that the literature on involuntary hospitalization provides little evidence that commitment laws which would make involuntary treatment easier to impose would have the effect of reducing homelessness among the mentally ill.

The tension between libertarian and paternalistic views of the rights of homeless people is often apparent in practice when an involuntary admission is needed. Colleagues who are generally allies of the psychiatrist in bringing help to homeless people may become adversaries when involuntary treatment is proposed. The solution to this problem often lies in the doctor's role as teacher. Many individuals who work with homeless people have limited professional training, or have backgrounds in social sciences, with little appreciation of the realities of mental illness. Working together over a period of time, and helping them to understand concepts of disease in psychiatry will reduce misunderstanding and disagreement.

PROGRAMS, MODELS AND SERVICE SYSTEMS

Increasing Accessibility

Special programs are needed for homeless people because of accessibility problems with conventional services. One set of problems is within the person: a distaste for conventional clinical settings, an exaggerated fear of how they will be treated, or a level of disorganization that makes it difficult for the person to get to the treatment facility. A second set of factors relates to the service programs themselves. There may be reluctance on the part of providers to deal with dirty or bizarre individuals, or a concern that such clients might scare away others. A clinic or agency may be located in a neighborhood that is off the beaten track for homeless people, or the cost or the complexity of its intake and registration procedures may serve as a deterrent (Stark, 1992). A classic example of the latter occurred during the 1980s, when the application procedures for Supplemental Security Income (SSI) were made so complex that most mentally ill people could not complete them without considerable assistance. Under pressure from homeless advocates, the situation was remedied. Not only was the procedure simplified, but special staff from the Social Security Administration were trained to go out in the streets of some cities to assist homeless people in making application for SSI.

Programs should be situated in areas frequented by homeless people. Public transport should be available. Buildings should not be intimidating, as many hospitals are. Facilities should be comfortable and attractive, as an inducement to enter, and as an indication that homeless people are respected and that their dignity and comfort are of concern to the program providers. There should be signs to assist people to find the program, but they should be sufficiently discrete to avoid stigmatization. The availability of services should be publicized through all the available media. In particular, other agencies serving homeless people should be fully aware of the location and hours of availability of mental health services.

Linkage and Collaboration

An individual program generally is only able to provide a partial response to the treatment needs of homeless people. Thus, in light of the wide range of services needed by many homeless people, service providers must take advantage of community service systems that are already in place. It often requires great diplomacy and much hard work to establish linkages with other treatment or rehabilitation programs in the area so that, through active liaison, the combined resources can be mobilized when needed. Considerable effort often needs to go into advocacy and obtaining support from state or local health service administrators.

Dual Diagnosis

The treatment of people with both mental illness and substance abuse or dependence (Drake & Wallach, 1989) perplexes service providers in community psychiatry programs generally (Minkoff & Drake, 1991), but especially in those working with homeless people, where the rates of co-morbidity are so high (Table 1.1). The problems encountered in attempting to treat dually diagnosed persons are both clinical and organizational.

The clinical problems arise from the difficulty of dealing simultaneously with two types of disorder. The psychiatric treatment of schizophrenia, for example, will lead to a diminution or elimination of many of the symptoms of the disease. Rehabilitation of the person, however, requires a concerted effort on the part of the patient and the professionals to move him or her in the direction of independence and self-sufficiency. Substance abuse greatly impedes this process. Conversely, remaining drug and alcohol free is, for an addict, a considerable feat, requiring volition, persistence, resilience and a supportive milieu, all of which may be lacking for a mentally ill person, especially one who is homeless. When a person has both a mental illness and a substance use disorder, each condition undermines the treatment of the other. The organizational problems arise because of the traditional separation of substance abuse and mental illness treatment services. This separation is reflected at the federal level, where separate bureaucracies deal with these problems: the National Institute of Mental Health (NIMH), the National Institute on Alcoholism and Alcohol Abuse (NIAAA), the National Institute on Drug Abuse (NIDA), the Center for Mental Health Services (CMHS), the Center for Substance Abuse and Treatment (CSAT). This same separation is reflected in bureaucracies at state and local levels, so that planning and implementing services to bring together treatment for mental illness and substance abuse is often complex.

Traditional service systems, therefore, often provide separate services for substance abuse and mental illness treatment, and efforts may be made to enrol a patient in both. Most often these plans do not succeed, and it has been found that integrated treatment programs are most effective. Integrated programs provide treatment for mental illness and treatment for substance abuse simultaneously, in a coordinated fashion, in the same setting, by the same staff (Ridgely, 1991).

The problems associated with dual diagnosis are compounded when the person is homeless (Minkoff & Drake, 1992). Alcohol has traditionally had an important place in the lives of homeless people (Hopper, 1989) and, for example, insisting on abstinence from alcohol or drugs as a prerequisite for participation in treatment may be counter-productive. Treatment programs for homeless dually diagnosed individuals may have abstinence as a goal to be attained, but nevertheless may admit individuals who are still drinking or using drugs (Minkoff & Drake, 1992).

THE FUTURE

Those who engage in providing services for homeless people do so in the hope that their services will soon no longer be needed, because homelessness will cease to be a major problem in American society. However this hope seems increasingly naive. As the years pass, the numbers of homeless people seeking help from service agencies only increases. The enormous deficiency in the supply of housing in America will take decades to remedy. Public opinion is currently not supportive of significant increases in assistance to the poor. Education for the masses of young Americans is not fitting them well for employment in an increasingly technological employment market. In spite of widespread hope in the early 1990s, adequate health care will not be guaranteed to all citizens in the foreseeable future. Community mental health services still struggle, both conceptually and financially, to provide comprehensive services for the mentally ill in the post-institutional era. Homelessness will therefore continue to be a problem in America, especially for the mentally ill. New approaches to addressing the problems of homeless people with serious mental illnesses are still needed and new service models still need to be developed and tested.

Whether there is progress along these lines will depend upon there being sufficient political will to make it possible. For this reason, psychiatrists and others who are concerned about these issues must involve themselves in political advocacy and public education, in concert with other groups who are active in this field.

REFERENCES

Appelbaum, P.S. (1992). Legal aspects of clinical care for severely mentally ill, homeless persons. *Bulletin of the American Academy of Psychiatry and the Law* 20:455–473.

Appleby, L. & Desai, P. (1987). Residential Stability: a pespective on system imbalance. *American Journal of Orthopsychiatry* 57:515–524.

Ball, F.L.J. & Havassy, B.E. (1984). A survey of the problems and needs of homeless consumers of acute psychiatric services. *Hospital and Community Psychiatry* 35:97–99.

Bassuk, E.L., Rubin, L. & Lauriat, A.S. (1986). Characteristics of homeless sheltered families. *American Journal of Public Health* 76:1097–1101.

Billig, N. & Levinson, C. (1987). Homelessness and case management in Montgomery County, Maryland: a focus on chronic mental illness. *Psychosocial Rehabilitation Journal* 11:59–66.

Blackwell, B. *et al.* (1990). Psychiatric and mental health services. In Brickner, P.W. *et al.* (1990). *Under the Safety Net: the health and social welfare of the homeless in the United States.* New York: Norton.

Breakey, W.R. & Fischer, P.J. (1995). Mental illness and the continuum of residential stability. *Social Psychiatry and Psychiatric Epidemiology* 30:147–151.

Breakey, W.R., Fischer, P.J., Kramer, M., Nestadt, G., Romanoski, A.J., Ross, A., Royal, R.M. & Stine, O.C. (1989). Health and mental health problems of homeless men and women in Baltimore. *Journal of the American Medical Association* 262:1352–1357.

Brickner, P.W. *et al.* (1990). *Under the Safety Net: the health and social welfare of the homeless in the United States.* New York: Norton.

Burt, M.R. & Cohen, B.E. (1989). *America's Homeless.* Washington, D.C.: The Urban Institute.

Cohen, C.I. (1993). Poverty and the course of schizophrenia: implications for research and policy. *Hospital and Community Psychiatry* 44:951–958.

Cohen, N.L. & Marcos, L.R. (1986). Psychiatric care of the homeless mentally ill. *Psychiatric Annals* 16:729–732.

Dellon, E.S. (1995). "The Health of the Providence Area Homeless Population." Honors thesis in Health and Society, Brown University.

Drake, R.E. & Wallach, (1989). Substance abuse among the chronically mentally ill. *Hospital and Community Psychiatry* 40:1041–1045.

Drake, R.E. & Adler, D.A. (1984). Shelter is not enough: clinical work with the homeless mentally ill. In: Lamb, H.R. ed. *The Homeless Mentally Ill.* Washington: American Psychiatric Association.

Farr, R.K. (1986). A mental health treatment program for the homeless mentally ill in the Los Angeles Skid Row area. In: Jones, B.E., ed. *Treating the Homeless: Urban Psychiatry's Challenge.* Washington, D.C., American Psychiatric Press.

Farr, R.K., Koegel, P. & Burnam, A. (1986). *A study of homelessness and mental illness in the Skid Row area of Los Angeles.* Los Angeles County Department of Mental Health.

Fischer, P.J. (1990). Estimating prevalence of alcohol, drug and mental health problems in the contemporarty homeless population: A review of the literature. *Contemporary Drug Problems* 16(3):333–390.

Fischer, P.J. & Breakey, W.R. (1986). Homelessness and mental health: an overview. *International Journal of Mental Health* 14(4):6–41.

Fischer, P.J. & Breakey, W.R. (1991). The epidemiology of alcohol, drug and mental disorders among homeless persons. *American Psychologist* 46:1115–1128.

Gelberg, L. & Linn, L.S. (1989). Assessing the physical health status of homeless adults. *Journal of the American Medical Association* 262:1973–1979.

Goering, P.N. & Wasylenki, D. (1996). Case management. In Breakey, W.R. (ed.) *Integrated Mental Health Services: Modern Community Psychiatry.* New York: Oxford University Press.

Herman, D.B., Struening, E.L. & Barrow, S.M. (1993). Self-assessed need for mental health services among homeless adults. *Hospital and Community Psychiatry* 44:1181–1183.

Holzer, C.E., Shea, B.M., Swanson, J.W., Leaf, P.J., Myers, J.K., George, L, Weissman, M. & Bednarski, P. (1986). The increased risk for specific psychiatric disorders among persons of low socioeconomic status. *American Journal of Social Psychiatry* 6:259–271.

Hopper, K. (1989). Deviance and dwelling space: notes on the resettlement of homeless persons with alcohol and drug problems. *Contemporary Drug Problems* 16:391–414.

Institute of Medicine. (1988). *Homelessness, health and human needs.* Washington, DC: National Academy Press.

Jahiel, R.I. (Ed.) (1992). *Homelessness: a prevention-oriented approach.* Baltimore: Johns Hopkins University Press.

Lamb, H.R., Bachrach, L.L. & Kass, F.I. (Eds.) (1992). *Treating the Homeless Mentally Ill.* Washington, D.C.: American Psychiatric Association.

Lamb, H.R., Bachrach, L.L., Goldfinger, S.M. & Kass, F.I. (1992). Summary and Recommendations. In Lamb, H.R., Bachrach, L.L. & Kass, F.I. (Eds.): *Treating the Homeless Mentally Ill.* Washington, D.C.: American Psychiatric Association.

Lomas, E. (1992). Skid-Row based services for people who are homeless and mentally ill. In Jahiel, R.I. (Ed.): *Homelessness: a prevention-oriented approach.* Baltimore: Johns Hopkins University Press.

Minkoff, K. & Drake, R.E. (1991). *Dual Diagnosis of major mental Illness and Substance Disorder.* San Francisco: Jossey-Bass.

Minkoff, K. & Drake, R.E. (1992). Homeless and dual diagnosis. In Lamb, H.R., Bachrach, L.L. & Kass, F.I. (Eds.): *Treating the Homeless Mentally Ill.* Washington, D.C.: American Psychiatric Association.

Ovrebo, B. (1992). Understanding the needs of homeless and near-homeless people. In Jahiel, R.I.: *Homelessness: a prevention-oriented approach.* Baltimore: Johns Hopkins University Press.

Reich, R. & Siegel, L. (1978). The emergence of the Bowery as a psychiatric dumping ground. *Psychiatric Quarterly* 50:191–

Ridgely, M.S. (1991). Creating integrated programs for severely mentally ill persons with substance disorders. In Minkoff, K. & Drake, R.E.: *Dual Diagnosis of major mental Illness and Substance Disorder.* San Francisco: Jossey-Bass.

Robertson, M.J. & Greenblatt, M. (Eds.) (1992). *Homelessness: a national perspective.* New York: Plenum Press.

Smith, E.M., North, C.S. & Spitznagel, E.L. (1992). A systematic study of mental illness, substance abuse and treatment in 600 homeless men. *Annals of Clinical Psychiatry* 4:111–120.

Smith, E.M., North, C.S. & Spitznagel, E.L. (1993). Alcohol, drugs and psychiatric comorbidity among homeless women: an epidemiological study. *Journal of Clinical Psychiatry* 54:82–87.

Spitzer, R.L., Cohen, Miller, J.D. & Endicott, J. (1969). The Psychiatric status of 100 men in skid row. *International Journal of Social Psychiatry* 15:230–234.

Stark, I. (1992). Barriers to health care for homeless people. In Jahiel, R.I.: *Homelessness: a prevention-oriented approach.* Baltimore: Johns Hopkins University Press.

Surber, R.W., Dwyer, E., Ryan, K.J., Goldfinger, S.M. & Kelly, J.T. (1988). Medical and psychiatric needs of the homeless. *Social Work* 33:116–119.

Susser, E., Valencia, E., Conover, S. (1993). Prevalence of HIV infection among psychiatric patients in a New York City men's shelter. *American Journal of Public Health* 83:568–570.

Susser, E., Struening, E.L. & Conover, S. (1989). Psychiatric problems in homeless men. *Archives of General Psychiatry* 46:845–850.

Susser, E., Valencia, E. & Goldfinger, S.M. (1992). Clinical care of homeless mentally ill individuals: strategies and adaptations. In Lamb, H.R., Bachrach, L.L. & Kass, F.I. (Eds.): *Treating the Homeless Mentally Ill.* Washington, D.C.: American Psychiatric Association.

Swayse, F.V. (1992). Clinical case management with the homeless mentally ill. In Lamb, H.R., Bachrach, L.L. & Kass, F.I. (Eds.): *Treating the Homeless Mentally Ill.* Washington, D.C.: American Psychiatric Association.

Tessler, R.C. & Dennis, D.L. (1989). *A synthesis of NIMH-funded research concerning persons who are homeless and mentally ill.* Rockville, Md.: National Institute of Mental Health.

Van Tosh, L. (1993). *Working for a change: Employment of consumers/survivors in the design and provision of services for persons who are homeless and mentally disabled.* Rockville, Maryland: Center for Mental Health Services.

Wright, J.D. & Weber, E. (1987). *Homelessness and Health.* Washington, D.C.: McGraw-Hill.

2

The Federal Role in Developing Solutions for Societal Problems

**ROGER B. STRAW, IRENE S. LEVINE and
FRED C. OSHER**

In the era of "reinventing government" and health care reform, questions are increasingly being raised about what role the Federal government should play in addressing societal problems. Such concerns have been debated for decades. At one pole are those who adopt the view that the Federal government should have no role in this arena; at the opposite pole are those who see social research and social policy as areas in which the Federal government is uniquely positioned to act, with the aim of helping the nation as a whole grapple with the major issues it confronts. The thesis of this chapter is that the Federal government can have an important role in supporting research and demonstration programs, 1) to generate knowledge about the effectiveness of client and system level interventions, 2) to disseminate these findings, and 3) to stimulate the adoption (or adaptation) of those approaches in community settings.

This chapter describes an approach utilized by federal policy makers, working collaboratively with researchers, providers, consumers and state and local officials, to find solutions to one of the most complex and vexing problems facing our society – homelessness among persons with severe mental illnesses. The federal McKinney homeless research demonstrations described in this volume are one phase in a systematic effort to develop effective service interventions for homeless persons with severe mental illnesses.

THE APPROACH

This approach has, as its basis, an iterative process of hypothesis generation, rigorous testing, and refinement of potential solutions, with the goal of identifying effective and well-defined interventions. This iterative process has three phases:

Phase I: Problem Identification through Epidemiological and Descriptive Research,

Phase II: Program Development through Exploratory (Services) Demonstrations,

Phase III: Testing and Refinement through Confirmatory (Research) Demonstrations.

Phase I begins with descriptive studies to identify the nature of an emerging social problem, examining both individual and system-level factors. These may include ethnographic and epidemiological studies of the population, studies of service needs and use of services, and studies of service systems. Phase II involves studying existing program models or the design and implementation of new programs to serve the population, based on the best available information (including descriptive studies and clinical knowledge). This information gathering on early program models is often referred to as a service demonstration, although *exploratory demonstration* is probably more descriptive of the purpose. Based on evidence of potential effectiveness from evaluations of service demonstrations, rigorous tests of the effectiveness of well-defined program models can occur. These Phase III studies have been referred to as research demonstrations although *confirmatory demonstrations* is, again, more descriptive of the purpose.

Once the effectiveness of particular models is established, planned replication of the models in new sites should be done. As the proven models are replicated in new sites, continued evaluation of program implementation and outcomes is required to ensure that modifications of the program model are identified, related changes in effectiveness, if any, are observed, and longitudinal outcomes are documented. To examine generalizability, variations on the basic program model can be studied systematically and their effects on outcomes documented. Unfortunately, federal demonstration programs focused on homeless persons with mental illnesses have not yet had the opportunity to explore replication in a systematic way.

Parallel to this strategy for the systematic generation of knowledge must be a commitment to the regular dissemination of findings to the broader practice community so that new knowledge can begin to influence program design and implementation at the earliest possible time. It is important to generate regular reports of progress and share interim findings so that the field is aware of work that is underway. These findings should be disseminated widely through a range of mechanisms, including reports and technical assistance as well as seed money for implementation, if it is available. The impact of these dissemination efforts on adoption of the proven models needs to be assessed on a regular basis so that efforts can be directed toward the more effective strategies.

HOMELESSNESS AND MENTAL ILLNESS

Fifteen years ago, Kim Hopper and Ellen Baxter, who are known nationally for their research and advocacy, documented the new face of homeless persons emerging on New York City streets which now included those disabled by mental illnesses, in a seminal piece for the Community Service Society entitled *Private Lives/Public Spaces* (Baxter & Hopper, 1981). They helped raise the consciousness of the public by better identifying a problem that was prevalent across the nation. A flurry of reports followed in both print and broadcast media.

In response to increasing popular and academic concern, the Federal government (through the efforts of the National Institute of Mental Health [NIMH], and more recently the Center for Mental Health Services [CMHS], embarked upon a research and demonstration program that has now spanned nearly 13 years and which has had a significant impact upon the way in which the mental health field views the problems of homelessness among persons with severe mental illnesses. This effort exemplifies a systematic approach to the design, implementation, and evaluation of a national demonstration program.

Phase I – Problem Identification Through Epidemiological and Descriptive Research

Beginning in 1982 and continuing until the present, the Federal government (through the National Institute of Mental Health) has awarded traditional competitive research grants to investigators to describe both the nature and extent of homelessness among persons with severe mental illnesses and the prevalence of mental illnesses among the homeless population. Initially, researchers had a difficult time developing successful applications focused on this topic. Typically, they met complex methodological, funding, and administrative barriers that needed to be overcome. For example, NIMH review committees were quite skeptical in their judgments about the significance and feasibility of research on homeless persons. In addition, they lacked background or expertise in the substantive area; as a result, the committee had to rely on more junior reviewers. These reviewers typically had limited experience in the review process and tended to be overly critical of their colleagues' proposals. To overcome these barriers, the NIMH leadership had to be convinced that an investment in addressing the meaningful and important questions of the relationship between severe mental illness and homelessness was needed. That investment included the education of potential investigators and review committees and the examination of NIMH funding priorities.

NIMH made its first competitive homelessness-related grant award in 1982 to William Breakey and Pamela Fischer of Johns Hopkins University. This successful effort documented the high prevalence of mental illness among homeless persons at the same time that the country was becoming increasingly aware of the presence of persons without adequate shelter – the "new homeless." Shortly thereafter, additional grants were awarded to other investigators to extend these results into other regions of the country and to gather critical data that could be used to inform service providers and policy-makers, and to develop more sophisticated research studies. These early studies and their results are summarized in *Two generations of NIMH-funded research on Homelessness and Mental Illness: 1982–1990* (National Institute of Mental Health, 1991). Before this time, State officials were reluctant, at best, to acknowledge the relationship between vicissitudes in public mental health policy and the emergence of homelessness. The NIMH data were telling and changed the nature of public discourse over the coming years.

During this same period, NIMH also funded a number of modest projects focused on identifying the service needs of homeless mentally ill persons. One particularly noteworthy initiative involved an American Psychiatric Association (APA) study of programs serving homeless mentally ill people. NIMH provided funds to the APA Task Force on the Homeless Mentally Ill to survey existing programs serving the population. These included both shelters and mental health programs. During a visit to New York City in 1983, one member of the site team was so viscerally moved by the sight of untreated mentally ill individuals at the Third Street Shelter that she had to leave the shelter and could not complete the visit. No one on the team was untouched by what they had seen and less than one year later, the Association produced a cogent and moving report, *The Homeless Mentally Ill* (American Psychiatric Association, 1984). Psychiatric leadership had now spoken: Any response to homelessness must necessarily entail housing, treatment, and social welfare considerations.

This early work set the stage for a dramatic change in the climate for homelessness research. In 1989, Lewis L. Judd, M.D. became Director of NIMH. Recognizing the critical importance of addressing this issue, Dr. Judd asked Irene Levine, Ph.D. to establish an office, reporting directly to the NIMH Director, to coordinate an expanded program of research, policy, and technical assistance activities focused on homelessness and severe mental illness. During an era of austere federal resources, new staff were also allocated to the program. A number of the individuals recruited to fill these positions have continued to make significant contributions to homelessness research and policy, including Debra Rog, Ph.D., now at Vanderbilt University and John Buckner, Ph.D., now with the Better Homes Foundation.

However, more importantly, Dr. Judd committed to set aside a sizeable pool of discretionary funds to jump-start research in this area. A new program announcement was developed to stimulate interest in the field. Needless to say, the availability of funds and

NIMH attention to the importance of the issue greatly accelerated both the quality and pace of research. Experienced researchers now had an incentive to engage in this relatively new and complex field of inquiry.

Ten research studies were funded in the initial year of the program announcement to expand understanding of the epidemiology of the homeless population and to study the reasons for entry into and exit from homelessness. Since then, NIMH has continued to fund research with an emphasis on understanding the dynamics of homelessness among particular segments of the population, including children and youth, families, minorities, persons involved with the criminal justice system, and persons with co-occurring mental illnesses and substance use disorders.

Phase II – Exploratory (Services) Demonstrations Program Development

With mounting congressional and public concern about homelessness, the Community Support Program (CSP) at NIMH issued an announcement in Fiscal Year 1986 that designated homeless persons with severe mental illnesses as a priority population for CSP service demonstrations. Coordination with other health and human service agencies and outreach to homeless individuals living in streets, shelters, and public transportation settings were among the important issues that applicants were expected to address. CSP funded fourteen projects that represented a wide variety of state-of-the-art approaches to serving homeless persons, including:

- assertive outreach in non-traditional settings;
- crisis intervention in shelters;
- case management on the streets;
- employment of paraprofessional or formerly homeless persons to provide services; and
- specialized housing arrangements, such as crisis residences and transitional housing.

In July 1987, Congress enacted the Stewart B. McKinney Homeless Assistance Act (P.L. 100-77) to establish a range of programs to assist the growing numbers of citizens experiencing homelessness. Contained in the Act were special provisions supporting further research on homelessness and severe mental illness as well as a new $30 million formula grant program called the Mental Health Services for the Homeless Block Grant. This block grant was subsequently renamed Projects for Assistance in the Transition from Homelessness (PATH). Much of the language and intent of the Act's mental health provisions relied on early NIMH research and data and on interim findings from demonstration projects discussed above.

Section 612 of the McKinney Act authorized Community Mental Health Services Demonstration Projects for Homeless Individuals

Who Are Chronically Mentally Ill. This new funding provided a mechanism for exploring the hypothesis that effective interventions would require comprehensive, coordinated mental health & support services. Using the Congressional appropriation of $9.3 million over two years, NIMH made awards to nine projects located in Chicago, Illinois; New York, New York; Flint/Ann Arbor, Michigan; Columbia, South Carolina; Portland, Oregon; Miami, Florida; Nashville, Tennessee; Cleveland, Ohio; and Richmond, Virginia. Seven of the nine projects also received a third year of funding, totaling an additional $4.6 million.

The projects were required to provide a package of services that included:

• outreach to homeless adults with severe mental illness in non-traditional settings;

• long-term, intensive case management;

• mental health treatment;

• supportive living programs; and

• management and administrative activities to integrate the services together into a comprehensive system of care.

In terms of evaluation, the projects were required to conduct an implementation and outcome evaluation and to cooperate with a national evaluation. Individual project evaluations were focused on describing the individuals served, services received, and client outcomes. The projects did not, as a general rule, have comparison or control groups. The national evaluation developed logic models for each of the projects and assessed the implementation of the projects through site visits and collateral materials (Abt Associates, 1991). An originally planned cross-site outcome evaluation was cancelled because of limited comparability across the projects and the limited client-level outcome data that was being collected.

The findings of the service demonstrations indicated that comprehensive supportive services were vital but that, in addition, access to permanent housing needed to be included in programs if they ultimately were to be successful. The potency of this finding bolstered the efforts of mental health policy-makers to solidify participation and fiscal support from the Department of Housing and Urban Development to its next generation of homeless demonstration projects. In addition, stronger evidence of positive outcomes was needed, as was further knowledge about the types of permanent housing required by homeless persons with severe mental illness.

Phase III – Testing and Refinement through Confirmatory (Research) Demonstration

In fiscal year 1990, Congress reauthorized the McKinney Act and appropriated $6 million to support a new set of demonstration projects for homeless persons with severe mental illnesses. Through a newly-developed Memorandum of Understanding between the U.S. Departments of Housing and Urban Development (HUD) and Health and Human Services, HUD contributed an additional $10 million of housing assistance over a 3 year period. The Memorandum acknowledged the necessity of links among clinical, supportive, and housing services. In keeping with the Memorandum, NIMH released a new Request for Applications in Spring, 1990. To compete successfully for funding, applicants had to propose clear hypotheses to be tested, a service program consistent with previous service demonstration findings, and a rigorous evaluation design.

Both implementation and outcome evaluations were required. The implementation evaluations were expected to describe client characteristics, provide information on the nature and characteristics of the mental health treatment, supportive services, and housing being provided, and assess whether the project was implemented as conceived. The outcome evaluations were designed to assess the effectiveness of project interventions through use of randomized control or comparison groups. Outcome evaluations addressed the extent to which program goals were met; whether the interventions were differentially effective in serving different subpopulations; and what factors are associated with effectiveness.

In September, 1990, the six teams of seasoned investigators, each of which has contributed a chapter to this book, were competitively selected to begin a methodologically sophisticated three-year program to test the effectiveness of a variety of approaches to providing mental health treatment, housing, and support services to homeless adults with severe mental illnesses. The principal investigators of the projects were nationally known and respected researchers and clinicians in the field of mental health services research. Within every project, the interdisciplinary research team included multiple institutional collaborators or co-investigators. As a group, these projects represent the first longitudinal, experimentally designed studies of housing and service interventions for homeless people with severe mental illnesses.

The implementation and evaluation of large demonstration projects in applied settings is extremely difficult. Occasionally, the difficulties are severe enough that research integrity is severely compromised and a project cannot accomplish its original research objectives. Unfortunately, one of the projects in this group had to be dropped after two years of funding because difficulties were encountered in implementing both the service program and the research component of the demonstration.

With Federal support, the principal investigators met as a group several times each year to review progress, make presentations at professional meetings, and develop cross-site analyses and publications. As a result of their commitment and interaction, a number of collaborative efforts have been undertaken. The first of these was an agreement to use a set of common measures that would allow the researchers to compare the effectiveness of interventions across projects more directly and to identify similar elements that help them achieve project goals and explain client outcomes. Common measures were used for the following domains: demographics, history of homelessness, residential stability, income and entitlements, quality of life (including living arrangements, finances, family/ social relationships, etc.), psychiatric symptomatology, and general health status. In addition, all five projects used the same measure of drug and alcohol dependence, the Addiction Severity Index, and four of the five projects used a common measure of psychiatric diagnosis, the Structured Clinical Interview for *DSM-III-R* (SCID). The one project not using the SCID (in San Diego) used the Diagnostic Interview Schedule (DIS) to make psychiatric diagnoses.

Initially within NIMH, and later in CMHS, funding for these projects over the subsequent three year period totaled $26.8 million (including the more than $10 million in housing assistance contributed by HUD). Interim findings from this program have been published in *Making a Difference* (Center for Mental Health Services, 1994)[1]. Although Federal funding of the studies is now complete, the researchers are continuing to analyze the data from their individual studies and publish the results. The data from the studies has also been combined into a pooled data set that is being used by the group of investigators to explore specific questions that could not be studied in any individual study. This work also continues and will be published over the next couple of years.

Further Refinement of Program Models

The projects described in this volume are focused primarily on the delivery and integration of services at the client level. During the implementation of the projects, observations suggested that fragmentation at the system level had a powerful effect on service delivery and client outcomes. These impressions were brought to the attention of the Federal Task Force on Homelessness and Severe Mental Illness which was charged with the task of developing policies to end homelessness among persons with severe mental illnesses. In the Task Force's report, *Outcasts on Main Street*, one of the principal recommendations was to develop a demonstration program focused on systems integration (Federal Task Force on Homelessness and Severe Mental Illness, 1992). In response to this recommendation, the Center for Mental Health Services used consolidated McKinney demonstration appropriations to develop a new program entitled Access to Community Care and Effective Services and Supports (ACCESS). Grants were awarded to nine states under this initiative in September, 1993. ACCESS is comparing the effectiveness of systems integration strategies combined with enhancements of services with simply enhancing the availability of appropriate services for homeless persons with severe mental illness.

A second major area of concern identified by the McKinney projects described in this volume, as well as others in the field, was the difficulty in serving homeless individuals with co-occurring mental and addictive disorders. There was general agreement that a more exploratory level of inquiry was needed to examine a range of potentially effective approaches to serving this subpopulation. As a result, the Center for Mental Health Services and the Center for Substance Abuse Treatment are co-sponsoring a demonstration program that will result in a set of treatment manuals based on existing service programs for the target population as well as preliminary evaluation data on the effectiveness of six of the most promising models of care.

Ongoing Dissemination of Findings

While the opportunity to develop demonstrations for the express purpose of replicating and disseminating particular models of care has not yet occurred, the Federal government continues to synthesize and disseminate the knowledge gained from this program of studies to service providers, policy makers, and researchers. By the late 1980s, the meetings and associated publications of staff and researchers sponsored by NIMH offered the field the first empirical evidence on the nature and extent of the problem of homelessness and the role of severe mental illness in the overall problem. Our early understanding of the extent of severe mental illness, substance abuse, and physical health needs in the homeless population, their involvement with the criminal justice and mental health systems, and the lack of income despite eligibility for public benefit programs, were recorded in a series of publications based on these meetings (Tessler and Dennis, 1989).

To assure ongoing collection, synthesis, and dissemination of research findings and information, NIMH established a clearinghouse dedicated to accumulating published and unpublished material related to homelessness and severe mental illness and producing syntheses of the growing knowledge base for the provider and consumer communities. This clearinghouse is known as the National Resource Center on Homelessness and Mental Illness. One of the first syntheses produced by the National Resource Center was *Two Generations of NIMH-funded Research on Homelessness and Mental Illness: 1982–1990* (National Institute for Mental Health, 1991). This monograph provided needed information to the field on the findings of the early research studies to the field at a time when it was very difficult to access the growing body of knowledge. Since then, the National Resource Center has continued to produce timely materials that synthesize the existing knowledge base such as *Making a Difference* (Center for Mental Health Services, 1994).

In addition, a variety of other technical assistance contracts have used the materials developed in these activities to directly inform service providers about the findings of the demonstration work. For example, CMHS supported technical assistance contracts for the PATH formula grant and Community Mental Health Services Block Grant programs that distribute information about state-of-the-art programming for this underserved population. CMHS also sponsors a broader mental health information clearinghouse that distributes this information to a wide variety of individuals and organizations with interests in mental health programs.

CONCLUSIONS

The evolving approach for addressing societal problems described in this chapter has been highly successful in moving researchers, service providers, and policy-makers relatively quickly from the identification of an emergent issue to a set of successful program models that are gaining increased acceptance in the mental health service community. We believe that this success is due in no small part to the Federal support for the systematic application of sound research and evaluation principles to the description of the problem and subsequent development and testing of alternative models for alleviating the problem.

There are impediments in the Federal system to conducting a systematic program of research and demonstrations but they are not insurmountable. Too often, research focuses on individual projects rather than on multi-year, multi-project research agendas that "add up to something." There is often reluctance, for example, to make relatively long-term investments in programmatic research and evaluation that extend beyond the term of one administration. Recent trends in the Federal government do not bode well for this type of approach. "Reinventing government", with its focus on customer service, may make it difficult to justify activities that do not immediately benefit the "customer". The Government Performance and Results Act, with its requirements to show annual progress toward quantifiable objectives, may push organizations toward short-term objectives at the expense of long-term solutions. Downsizing of the Federal workforce may affect the ability of organizations to devote staff to activities such as these. On the other hand, a renewed interest in re-examining the Federal role in social programs could lead to stronger political support for the use of limited available resources in research and evaluation.

We believe strongly that the approach described here is highly generalizable to other problems, and that the methods described above can be replicated in any number of specific areas, such as welfare reform. The resources required to do so, both in terms of program funds and federal staff, are small, relative to total federal expenditures to address most social problems; the findings from systematic research, on the other hand, can play a large part in planning successful programs.

REFERENCES

Abt Associates (1991). *Implementation evaluation report*. Cambridge, MA: Abt Associates, Inc.

American Psychiatric Association (1984). *The Homeless Mentally Ill: A Task Force Report of the American Psychiatric Association*. Washington, D.C.: American Psychiatric Association.

Baxter, E. & Hopper, K. (1981). *Private lives, public spaces: Homeless adults on the streets of New York City*. New York: Community Service Society.

Center for Mental Health Services (1994). *Making a Difference: Interim Status Report of the McKinney Research Demonstration Program for Homeless Mentally Ill Adults.* Rockville, MD: Center for Mental Health Services.

Federal Task Force on Homelessness and Severe Mental Illness (1992). *Outcasts on Main Street: Report of the Federal Task Force on Homelessness and Severe Mental Illness.* Washington, DC: Interagency Council on the Homeless.

National Institute of Mental Health (1991). *Two generations of NIMH-funded research on Homelessness and Mental Illness: 1982–1990.* Rockville, MD: National Institute of Mental Health.

ENDNOTE

1. Copies of *Making a Difference* may be obtained from the National Resource Center on Homelessness and Mental Illness at (800) 444-7415.

3

Housing Persons who are Homeless and Mentally Ill: Independent Living or Evolving Consumer Households?

STEPHEN M. GOLDFINGER, RUSSELL K. SCHUTT, GEORGE S. TOLOMICZENKO, WINSTON M. TURNER, NORMA WARE, WALTER E. PENK, MARK S. ABLEMAN, TARA L. AVRUSKIN, JOSHUA BRESLAU, BRINA CAPLAN, BARBARA DICKEY, OLINDA GONZALEZ, BYRON GOOD, SONDRA HELLMAN, SUSAN LEE, MARTHA O'BRYAN and LARRY J. SEIDMAN

In spite of a growing literature on people who are homeless and mentally ill, little systematic evidence is available on how best to meet their housing and service needs. Research indicates that simultaneous provision of housing and support services may improve residential stability, health, and functioning of formerly homeless mentally ill persons. However, prior studies have not identified either the type of housing that is most effective nor the subgroups that are most likely to benefit from any particular combination of housing and services. This chapter describes an evaluation of two models of housing provision, one in which individuals who are mentally ill and have been homeless are supported in traditionally managed housing arrangements and another in which the consumers themselves assume control of the housing arrangement.

HOUSING MODELS AND HOUSING PREFERENCES

Different mental health professionals have recommended a variety of housing models for homeless mentally ill persons. These include: independent apartments (Blanch *et al.*, 1988; Ridgway, *et al.*,1988), housing with supportive services (Allard & Carling, 1986; Axelrod & Toff, 1987), and a continuum of housing alternatives of decreasing service intensity (Bassuk & Lamb, 1986; Lamb, 1984). Prior research fails to provide much guidance: it appears that housing with some service supports can improve some outcomes for some homeless mentally ill persons, but the merits of alternative housing models have not been systematically evaluated (Lipton *et al.*, 1988; Rosenheck *et al.*, 1989).

Research also has been scant on what type of housing homeless mentally ill persons *want*, although extant studies indicate a marked preference for independent living (Barrow *et al.*, 1989; Blanch *et al.*, 1988; Carling, 1990; Elliott *et al.*, 1990; Goering *et al.*, 1990; Thomas, 1987). Consumer advocates often criticize group homes for the extent to which they regulate residents' lives, the fact that they are transitional in nature, and that clients are not allowed to select their own roommates. In sum, these advocates contend that group homes fail to prepare clients adequately for independent living (Ridgway *et al.*, 1988). Whether implementing a policy consistent with such consumer preferences would affect residential tenure either positively or negatively has yet to be determined (Depp *et al.*, 1983; Levine & Parrish, 1986; Susser *et al.*, 1990).

Homelessness and Housing in Boston

Although metropolitan Boston in many respects provided greater access to shelters and services than many American cities, permanent housing was in short supply. For those with mental illness among the homeless population, the case may have been even worse. Both generic and specialized mental health shelters, initially set up as "emergency" or "brief transitional" accommodations, frequently were unable to secure appropriate housing for their residents. Designed for stays to be measured in weeks and months, in 1990 many individuals had lived in these settings for almost a decade. With the economic declines of the late 1980s and the fiscal "belt tightening" which followed, little new housing was to be funded. An array of staffed community-based group residences were tied to each of the local mental health centers, but waiting lists were long and individuals coming from inpatient psychiatric services had priority for housing. Although independent apartments were also available to the mental health centers, center staff operated with the working assumption held by many clinician that in order to develop community-based living skills, severely and persistently mentally ill individuals should progress through an ordered series of group residences to demonstrate that they can manage adequately on their own in independent apartments.

The availability of HUD funding for housing tied to McKinney Demonstration Projects (Center for Mental Health Services, 1994) resulted in widespread administrative support for a Boston McKinney Research Demonstration application. Although there was great ambivalence both about group homes "run" by consumers, and about the risks attendant on randomly assigning severely mentally ill individuals to independent living, the possibility of establishing 118 new units of housing was a powerful motivator.

THE BOSTON MCKINNEY PROJECT

The Boston Research Demonstration Project developed two distinct residential alternatives: Evolving Consumer Households (ECH) and Independent Living (IL). Both models were designed to maximize the likelihood of participant success, but the principal hypothesis for the study was that the ECH model would result in better outcomes.

The Evolving Consumer Household Model

Seven renovated or newly constructed houses provided a total of 63 beds in Evolving Consumer Households. Building occupancy ranged from 5 to 10 tenants, with virtually all tenants in separate bedrooms (a few homes had one two-bedded room). The houses provided shared living, dining, recreational and kitchen facilities. Tenants were free to share as much or as little of these facilities as they wished; food could be kept separately or communally, as they desired. The houses began with around the clock staffing, generally with 2–3 staff on during the day and evening, and one staff on duty and awake at night.

A philosophy of consumer empowerment seemed the likely antidote to the ingrained, institutional dependence so well documented among those with chronic mental illnesses. Severely mentally ill homeless individuals are traditionally viewed as recidivists who frequently return to homelessness and to the shelters from which others have worked so hard to enable their departure. Once housed, these men and women are often expected to "fail" in their placements and to become homeless once again.

The ECH model was meant to strike the most appropriate balance between consumers' demands for greater autonomy and clinicians' concerns about the important role of social support in minimizing the risk of housing loss. We agreed with consumers that they should be able to live independently, but believed that they would require support while they learned (or relearned) how to do so. We objected to the requirement that consumers move through a succession of residences in order to gain independence. Instead, we felt that consumers would do best in one residence where support services would be withdrawn gradually over time. As a result, Evolving Consumer Households were designed so that they began with 24-hour staffing, but were expected to be "taken over" gradually by the consumers living in them. These consumer-tenants were not expected to move; rather, staff were asked to leave as consumers learned to take responsibility for their own affairs.

In addition to reducing disruptions in living arrangements, we believed that the ECH approach would have several other distinct advantages over other models for developing client autonomy. First, this model would provide a more realistic and broadly applicable approach to housing than either independent apartments or traditional group homes. The initial presence of 24-hour staff would offer support and supervision required for some individuals whose clinical condition might otherwise preclude their placement in independent apartments. Rather than requiring autonomous functioning as a *pre-condition* for community placement, these households allow site-specific skills and abilities necessary for independent living to evolve over time.

Two fundamental principles of house management represented this philosophy:

1) The locus of control for operating each residence should be centered on the consumer residents. They, collectively, should help set household routine, establish staff priorities, determine the degree and nature of services they desire, and in collaboration with each residence's program director, set the policies and procedures for their home.

2) The goal of the residence, established at the outset, was to initiate and foster an evolving process toward enabling housed subjects to take over all staff functions. As ECH residents felt both willing and able, they were expected to systematically assume household responsibilities initially held by paid staff. Thus, for example, early on, consumers began to manage such functions as shopping, cleaning and preparing meals. A second tier of possible responsibilities included managing their own night-time coverage, purchasing supplies, arranging for household repairs, and paying for utilities and other household expenses.

Empowerment required that the well-meant and directive intentions of the staff to prevent, avoid, and/or to resolve problems had to be held in check. Housing staff were reminded regularly to teach clients to do for themselves. The successful implementation of an empowerment philosophy within an intervention program also required that someone take responsibility for its consistent enforcement. In the Boston project, this "consumer's watch" function was maintained by a former teacher experienced in work with mentally ill people (Brooks) who embraced the empowerment philosophy, created training curricula for both staff and clients, and consistently monitored staff behavior and attitudes.

Second, a possible shortcoming of independent apartments as permanent housing is their tendency to foster isolation and alienation from others – a tendency that is exacerbated in a population whose psychiatric symptoms (including paranoia, apathy, anhedonia or delusional thought) often lead to social withdrawal

(Mulkern *et al.*, 1986; Fischer & Breakey, 1986; Tessler & Dennis, 1989). The ECH approach was therefore designed to encourage supportive social relationships.

Finally, we believed that the group household approach would have several practical advantages: shared expenses, shared household tasks, and an enhanced quality of residence possible when renting multi-bedroom units.

The Independent Living Model

Fifty-five units of independent, single room occupancy accommodations, including both scattered-site apartments and single rooms in buildings with some communal space, were provided. Almost all of these were in public housing facilities run by the Boston Housing Authority. Initially, none of these units offered any on-site programming or resident clinical staff, although each building had a part-time coordinator who served as liaison between the Project, the building and the Department of Mental Health. At the recommendation of our consumer consultants, groups were offered every week or two, open to any residents of the building (or of nearby buildings) designed to offer social contact and some help with residential problem-solving. Study participants were not required to participate in treatment, although they were encouraged by their case managers to make use of CMHC clinical services appropriate to their clinical needs and level of functioning.

The Role of Case Management

Each participant in the project was assigned an intensive clinical case manager (ICCM) for the project's duration. ICCMs worked directly and intensively with a caseload of no more than 15 subjects (living in both housing settings) to ensure that gains in functioning were maximized and maintained. They also provided service brokerage functions, including assistance in obtaining entitlements, coordinating service components, and encouraging subject participation in rehabilitative and self-help programs. We believe that the use of intensive clinicial case managers ensured that consumers assigned to independent living did not fall through cracks in the service system and that all project participants could have access to assistance when they needed it.

THE RESEARCH DESIGN

Specific hypotheses were as follows:

1) Client outcomes would be more favorable in Evolving Consumer Households than in Independent Living situations;

2) Client outcomes would be more favorable when client's and clinician's choice of housing type match the housing type to which a client was randomly assigned.

In addition to these specific hypotheses, we sought to answer a number of related research questions, ranging from the descriptive ("What are the clinical, demographic, and functional descriptions of individuals currently living in the transitional shelter system?" and "What are the housing preferences of homeless mentally ill persons?") to the explanatory ("What individual characteristics predict better outcomes in group living situations?" and "How do social supports change after obtaining housing?"). Exploratory questions about the process of housing development were also addressed: "What is the process by which group homes can evolve into independent consumer-operated households?" "Can a model which fosters increasing consumer independence and management be replicated in multiple residences?"

The study focussed on outcome and process. We defined outcome operationally as client status at the end of the 18 month study period with respect to housing tenure, mental and physical health, social functioning, life satisfaction and substace abuse. To control for variables known to mediate these outcomes, we collected data on subject demographic and clinical history, diagnosis, neuropsychological functioning, and service use. Most measures were administered at baseline and then repeated at six month intervals. (The neuropsychological assessment battery and the Minnesota Multiphasic Personality Inventory, Second Edition were administered twice: at baseline and again after 15 months).

Special attention was given in the research design to the measurement and analysis of variables that we believed would influence both housing evolution and individual outcomes, including neuropsychological functioning, substance abuse, social support, and life skills. Supplementary studies allowed additional interviewing to measure subjects' personalities and their awareness of AIDS risks.

The process analysis was designed to monitor service delivery by case managers and to explore the development of the Evolving Consumer Households. An additional grant allowed collection of comprehensive data on subjects' use of hospital and other mental health services and calculation of the cost of these services.

The Intensive Clinicial Case Managers completed logs of their activities, indicating the time they spent with subjects on different service activities each week. On the same form, case managers reported what they had learned about subjects' use of services as well as subjects' residential status. The collection of these data at weekly intervals facilitated the detection of relocations, hospitalizations and elopements from the assigned housing sites. Every six months, ICCMs also completed a Life Skills Profile (Rosen *et al.*, 1989) for each subject.

We knew that the development of consumer-managed collective households was a sufficiently novel and unprecedented approach that we could not guarantee that all Evolving Consumer Households would move systematically and uniformly toward the goal of independence and tenant control. Studying the process of housing evolution of each of these "micro-cultures" became the responsiblity of a team of three anthropologists. Each ethnographer spent several days per week speaking with and observing tenants and staff in at least two group households. This work resulted in detailed notes on household evolution as well as identification of critical problems that required early intervention.

PROJECT IMPLEMENTATION

Implementing the project required obtaining access to suitable housing stock, refining plans for the Evolving Consumer Households, recruiting and orienting consumers, and training a case management staff.

Housing Development

The design, procurement and development of housing is never an easy task for a human service agency, especially when the intended residents are individuals who are handicapped by either physical or psychiatric conditions. The Boston McKinney project was only able to acquire sufficient housing for the study through cooperation of federal, state and local governments, local mental health providers, and the tenacious determination of the project staff.

The regional office of the Department of Mental Health (DMH) and the four existing Community Mental Health Centers (CMHCs) had demonstrated experience in developing independent apartments. The project co-investigator who oversaw the housing section of the Project for the Metro Boston Department of Mental Health (O'Bryan) secured access to individual apartments in HUD-financed elderly housing units throughout the city. Fifty five units of independent, single occupancy accommodations, including both scattered site apartments and single rooms in buildings with some communal space, were provided.

The providers responsible for the development of the ECHs all had longstanding experience in designing, implementing and operating a wide variety of community-based residential housing for the severely and persistently mentally ill. The Principal Investigator (Goldfinger), two co-investigators (O'Bryan & Hellman) and project clinical leadership (Abelman & Brooks) met regularly with housing agencies and worked with them in every step of the contract preparation for the sites. The staff for each new house were specifically recruited with the understanding that a fundamental task of their job was to insure their own obsolescence and transfer to another housing site. Project leadership also met with each house director to ensure understanding of the goals of the residential alternatives.

Consumer Consultants

Four past and current consumers actively involved in the development and management of consumer-run self-help programs served as project consultants. The consultant group met with ECH staff in a planning session prior to finalizing the residential program and then again after most staff were hired. These meetings provided an opportunity for staff and management to become familiar with existing examples of consumer-run self-help models, to work together with consumer experts in designing specific aspects of the ECH model, and to outline a structure where providers and consumers could, as colleagues, share their experiences and concerns. A fundamental goal of these sessions was to provide a shared vision of how these households could develop and to address possible barriers to effective implementation and strategies for overcoming them.

Subject Selection

Subjects were drawn from among homeless individuals with serious and persistent mental illnesses between the ages of 18 and 65 residing in Boston's three DMH transitional shelters. Each of the shelters' residents was assessed on his or her ability to remain safe if placed in an independent apartment. This assessment was performed by the Project's housing coordinator (Brooks) using current and prior psychiatric history. Shelter residents at imminent risk of dangerousness to self or others (e.g. threatening behavior, suicidality, fire setting, brain damage and other impairments which might lead to accidental misuse of stoves, matches, or cigarettes) were eliminated from current placement and re-evaluated six months later. All residents who passed this "safety screen" were referred to the Project Director and were informed of the nature of the project using a standard informed consent protocol.

Pre-move Preparation

Clients who consented to participate in the Project were interviewed at their shelters by Project research staff using an initial assessment schedule. Interview results were again reviewed with the Project Director to ensure that all study subjects were homeless, seriously mentally ill, had given informed and voluntary consent, and were safe. Eligible subjects entered a period of training and data collection prior to placement into housing. All subjects participated in a Housing Education Forum at the shelter, consisting of structured education groups designed to orient subjects to independent community living. Modeled on the groups developed by Andrea White (Susser *et al.*, 1990), the forums facilitated the discussion of advantages and disadvantages of various possible living situations. The goals and expectations of living in both independent apartments and evolving consumer homes were discussed. Thus, before data on individuals' housing preferences were collected, every effort was made to educate all subjects about the realities of living in the different housing options. Following a five week course of these didactic and interactive sessions, consumer housing preference information was collected.

During the period prior to their move, participants' housing needs were assessed by two independent clinical consultants. Gathering data from all available sources (shelter staff, case records, current therapists, and client interviews), each clinical consultant independently answered a range of questions about housing options and determined which of the two residential alternatives they believed most closely represented the ideal placement for the subject. The consultants also predicted how well each subject would do in different sites out of a spectrum of housing placement and clinical care options.

Case Management

Both ECH and IL subjects were followed by an individually-assigned ICCM. The pre-move preparation included regular meetings between subjects and their ICCMs. Skill training for shopping, food preparation, and mastering important public transportation routes was done. Visits to their new residence allowed subjects to become familiar with their assigned home and to "check out the neighborhood." Those assigned to ECHs were introduced to their new housemates and familiarized themselves with household routines. The process helped subjects who had lived in the transitional shelters for extended periods to manage transitions from old friendships or to maintain contacts.

Once placed in the residence, subjects were seen at least weekly by their ICCM. Contacts occurred within residences, at the Project offices, and in the subjects' neighborhoods or at the site of day activity programs. In addition, the local community mental health centers (CMHCs) and systems of services offered subjects an array of treatments – medication clinics, individual and group therapies, day programs for rehabilitation and social day activities and, if needed, crisis intervention and inpatient hospitalization. Subjects were encouraged to utilize appropriate services but informed that their housing and case management services were not contingent upon their doing so.

To assure uniformity in clinical stance and theoretical perspective, each ICCM met regularly with the Project Director or senior clinical supervisor for clinical and caseload supervision. In addition, the entire staff participated in regular weekly Project staff meetings. A clinically pragmatic style guided the project case management (Frances & Goldfinger, 1986; Goldfinger et al., 1990; Chafetz & Goldfinger, 1984; Harris & Bergman, 1987; Harris & Bachrach, 1988; Kanter, 1985).

Data Collection

Data collection began with initial baseline assessment of subjects after eligibility was determined. Subjects who enrolled were then randomly assigned to one of the housing conditions. Thereafter, data were collected from clients and ICCMs every six months from the date of entry into the study. Post-doctoral level psychologists (Tolomiczenko & Caplan) administered a Structured Clinical Interview for DSM-III-R (SCID) to provide an Axis I lifetime diagnosis at baseline and a battery of neuropsychological tests at baseline and at 15 months. All other data were collected by trained research assistants.

RESEARCH FINDINGS

The research has produced a comprehensive description of homeless mentally ill persons, a detailed exploration of the process of developing consumer-run housing, a systematic record of service delivery, and data on the effects of alternative housing models and the other factors that influence residential stability, health, functioning, and other outcomes.

Description of the Sample

The sample contained a somewhat higher proportion of women and whites and fewer veterans than most samples of the general homeless population. About one-third were women, almost half were from minority groups and 15% were veterans (see Table 3.1). Fifteen percent were employed (in part-time or "odd jobs" only). Only three percent were currently married and one-quarter were separated or divorced. About half had less than 12 years of schooling, while one in five had some college.

DSM-III-R lifetime diagnoses (as determined by the baseline SCID) for over half of the sample were within the schizophrenia-spectrum of disorders (a schizophrenia subtype or schizoaffective disorder). All but one subject had a major Axis I disorder. Baseline neuropsychological testing revealed many cognitive impairments. This was particularly true of the schizophrenia-spectrum subjects.

Most of the sample were current consumers of mental health services. Nine in ten were on psychotropic medication, 97% had been in outpatient treatment and 83% had been hospitalized for psychiatric problems – 28% more than five times and 45% within the last six months. About half of the sample initially described themselves as substance abusers – a proportion typical of studies of homeless mentally ill persons.

Among these homeless individuals, interest in moving out of the shelter into some type of housing was almost universal. When confronted with a choice of living in their own apartment or with a

Table 3.1. Sample Characteristics

Age	m = 37.6, s = 8.1
Gender (female)	29%
Race (African American)	41%
Veteran Status (veteran)	15%
Employment Status (employed)	15%
Marital Status:	
Never married	70%
Married	3%
Separated or Divorced	27%
Years of Schooling	
<12	49%
12	30%
>12	21%
Psychiatric Treatment:	
Currently Taking Medications	90%
Ever In Outpatient Treatment	97%
Ever Hospitalized	83%
Hospitalized More than 5 Times	28%
Hospitalized Within Last 6 Months	45%

group, respondents chose independent living by a wide margin, but many consumers were interested in having assistance from staff after moving into their own quarters. One-third clearly rejected staff help for anything but the most difficult problems (Schutt & Goldfinger, in press).

Subjects were randomly assigned to the two types of housing: sixty-three subjects were assigned to the ECHs and fifty-five were assigned to the ILs.

Outcomes

Service utilization: Case management time and detoxification admissions were recorded by the ICCMs weekly. Data on mental health treatment, including hospitalizations, were provided to the research staff by the providers – typically CMHC personnel. The Department of Mental Health inpatient files were also used to verify hospitalizations. For the 111 subjects for whom complete data are available for 18 months, we found that the total utilization of a particular service differed significantly only in time hospitalized for psychiatric reasons: ECH subjects averaged 15.8 days versus 27.9 days for IL subjects ($t = -1.90$, $p = 0.03$, one-tailed).

Residential status: Overall, subjects did very well in maintaining housing stability. While there was considerable movement during the project, a significant majority of the group were maintaining some type of community residential status by the end of the study. Of the 109 for whom housing data were available at 18 months, 88 (81%) were maintaining housing, 65 in their originally assigned housing site and the remaining 23 in other community housing. Of the remaining 21 subjects, 16 had returned to the shelter system, five were on the streets and one was in jail.

Differences between housing types in the frequency and duration of homelessness were not statistically significant, but all were in the predicted direction: ECH subjects had fewer episodes of homelessness and spent fewer days homeless. Among possible predictors of housing loss, substance abuse proved to be, by far, the most important.

Clinical and social indicators: Few clinical and social changes were noted between housing conditions, but there were some important changes over time and interactions with housing type. Quality of life measures were relatively invariant, although consumers in the ECHs were less satisfied than their IL counterparts with the degree of privacy in their housing. Neither self-reported symptoms of mental illness, nor perceived social support appeared to change over time or to differ between housing types.

Follow-up neuropsychological testing did reveal significant improvement in some areas, although the pattern of change was similar between the two housing interventions. Residential preferences also changed, although in interaction with substance abuse and type of housing. Consumers assigned to Evolving Consumer Households developed more liking for group living over time, but only if they were not substance abusers at baseline. Substance abusers were adamantly opposed to group living at baseline and remained so throughout the project.

Housing evolution: The transition from shelter living to ECH tenancy required a dramatic change in the quality of subjects' relationships. In contrast to the detached style of sociability that many shelter residents adopt and seem to prefer, ECH living requires that residents involve themselves with their peers. For example, as part of helping to prepare them for living as members of a group, staff encouraged tenants to learn techniques for resolving interpersonal conflicts by "confronting" the perpetrator of objectionable behaviors. These and other forms of increasing engagement with housemates – sharing meals, collecting money to pay joint household expenses – were viewed by staff as part of the development of a "sense of community." A sense of community among tenants was deemed critical to their eventual ability to maintain themselves in the house without on-site assistance (Ware *et al.*, 1992).

The ethnographic observers described the evolution process in the residences as a series of struggles. Staff struggled with tenants to show or convince them, for example, that the tenants were capable of assuming responsibility. Staff members also struggled internally and amongst themselves in their attempts to let go of traditional roles and attitudes and to create "new ways of being" with those they serve. The tenants themselves struggled with each other to find ways to resolve interpersonal conflicts and to share the management of the house equitably.

The staff's first significant encounter with the empowerment process usually came with the realization that they were expected to treat the residence as belonging to the tenants. This meant, among other things, spending time in the tenants' space only when needed or asked to by tenants. Responses ranged from good-willed and sincere attempts at cooperation to subtle (and less subtle) forms of resistance. In one house, where the "office" was on the third floor, a refrigerator, armchair and various other conveniences were installed and, except when they were involved in assisting or talking with tenants, staff spent their time there. In another, where staying in the office could mean crowding four or five people into a tiny space, staff tended to find reasons to leave – to smoke, to get a drink of water, or to ask tenants questions that "can't wait." At first staff voiced complaints of loneliness, or feelings of uselessness, or unfairness, while tenants reveled in their new-found authority, gleefully reminding staff of their responsibility to stay in the office and instructing them to return there at will. Over time, however, the social dynamics shifted. Tenants found themselves wandering into the office to talk to staff, inviting staff out to watch TV, and initiating contact in other ways. A new, perhaps somewhat more equal, form of staff-tenant relations gradually emerged.

The stress of living with adult roommates may be heightened for persons who have in various senses been socially isolated and who may also have difficulty in managing interpersonal relations. There were disputes – over keeping the bathrooms clean, over leaving dirty dishes in the sink, over borrowing money and bumming cigarettes, over playing the radio too loudly, over perceived insults, actual insults, misunderstandings. Tenants were confronted with the task of finding ways of getting along with each other in spite of objections to behavior, mistrust, and in some cases, active disapproval and dislike. Slowly, with difficulty, in collaboration with project staff, they developed informal and formal mechanisms for resolving or at least addressing differences and concerns.

One informal mechanism that evolved with support and encouragement from staff was bringing things up in meetings. "Bringing things up" meant communicating negative feelings about a housemate's behavior, for example, directly to the individual involved. Staff felt strongly that open airing of grievances would result in constructive change – behavior would be modified to accommodate to the needs and preferences of others and the group of individuals would transform itself into a community. Tenants, however, resisted, citing apprehensions about the negative consequences of direct confrontations with others. Gradually, however, they did bring things up – first obliquely, refraining from naming names, couching complaints in jokes – then more directly. Skills in negotiating, in compromising, increased (Ware et al., 1992).

When bringing things up was insufficient and tensions were running high, a more formal mechanism was sometimes invoked. Again with the help of project staff, tenants developed a system of communicating by letter. Together, they would agree on what they wanted to say and write it out in pen or pencil, with staff sometimes helping with the phrasing. Staff would then type the letter, the tenants would sign it, and one of them would, at an agreed-upon time, deliver it to the intended recipient. Most often the letter contained a series of requested changes in behavior, followed by an implicit or explicit reference to the consequences of failing to comply with the requests. In extreme cases, the consequences were defined as being asked to leave the residence. The following is an actual example:

Dear Billy,

Your behavior in this house does not meet the standards we have set for our household. We have discussed this formally at tenant meetings. If you want to continue to live here, you need to immediately change some of the things you do. They are as follows:

1. Respect the rule of no alcohol in the house.

2. Be respectful of other people.

3. Clean up after yourself.

4. Pay your share of the housefund without constant reminders.

5. Do not play loud music after 10:00 p.m.

6. Do not yell, or use profanity or threatening language.

We have requested program staff to help intervene. They are willing to meet with you to help you do the things that are required for you to stay here.

We are all grown-up people here. No one should be favored. Everyone should be treated equal.

We do not want you to lose your home here, but we can't stand the way you are treating us anymore.

Signed,

RESEARCH ISSUES FOR FUTURE PROJECTS

Data were collected successfully on a wide range of process issues and subject outcomes, but we encountered several problems that should be taken into account in future research.

Subject Recruitment and Retention

Although we had originally anticipated that attrition was going to be a significant problem, since prerequisites for our sample were histories of chronic homelessness and severe mental illness, in reality it was not. Of the 118 individuals who successfully moved into project-provided housing, only 9 were lost to 18-month follow-up. Four had died, three had moved out of state and two were excluded following randomization when a criminal record check precluded assignment. At each testing interval, some data points were lost because subjects were unavailable for testing or interviewing (e.g. three subjects were in jail and others episodically refused to be interviewed). This resulted in some differences in the number of data points at each interval and for each part of the test and interview protocol.

Measurement Issues

An important aspect of this research has been to demonstrate that these individuals are largely able to comply with the stress necessarily involved with a large battery of interviews and tests. Almost all were able to complete the basic interview package lasting three hours and a battery of cognitive tests which, on average, took two sittings, each of three hours duration, to complete. Most completed the 567-question MMPI-2 at baseline, although willingness to participate declined markedly in the follow-up interview – perhaps because many subjects were not assessed with a follow-up MMPI-2 questionnaire until after they had been told the project was over. Clients were reimbursed for their time in direct contact with research staff for interviews or testing at a rate of five dollars per hour.

Multiple methods: Self-report measures were inadequate as measures of two of our most significant areas of concern: substance abuse and housing status. In particular, substance use proved to be a difficult activity to measure accurately. We used both self-reports, the Addiction Severity Index and the SCID, and ratings by ICCMs. None of these sources could be relied on by itself, as many apparent substance abusers were identified with one instrument but not with another.

Two distinct measures of housing tenure were obtained. The first was the subjects' self-report of where they had lived during the six months prior to each follow-up interview. This measure captured the subjects' own perception of their housing stability during the project. Housing chronologies were also constructed using ICCM reports and, in general, there were strong correlations between self-report and observational data provided by the ICCMs, but self-reported time spent in categories of "housing" indicative of poor outcomes were typically underestimates of more accurate observer-collected data. This applied to time spent in detox programs, time hospitalized for psychiatric reasons and time homeless (living on the streets or in shelters).

Collecting provider data: Collection of process data was difficult and time consuming. ICCM logs provided important process data, but it was difficult to develop an adequate procedure for ensuring reliability over time and among case managers. Initial group meetings with ICCMs helped in tailoring our log form to the experiences of project ICCMs, but clinical staff turnover and inconsistent contact with the project research staff made it difficult to maintain standards. We did succeed in collecting comprehensive data on use of services outside of the project.

SERVICE ISSUES FOR FUTURE PROJECTS

Consumer Empowerment

One of the most interesting challenges of this project was the establishment of the housing itself using such a controversial housing model. How do you train staff to take a position in which they are expected to believe that, in essence, "My job is to make the clients in my house so empowered that they will lay me off and be able to manage without me."? The fundamental goal was to begin to teach people a way of existing in the community without needing staff support and to encourage tenants to make their own decisions. It is now abundantly clear that many more clinicians are in favor of empowerment as a concept than favor handing over their power!

"Empowerment" is a buzzword commonly used by clinicians, consumers and policy makers. In practice, however, letting someone else make a decision that you believe is really yours to make is a complicated achievement. "Empowered" clients initially behaved as passive inmates; it took months for many to use the open door and to see themselves as free to make their own decisions.

ECH staff were faced with questions such as what to do when residents decided that they were going to be serving wine and beer with dinner when half were substance abusing and all were mentally ill. The house staff actually thought this decision was quite reasonable, as long as behavior was under control and consistent with the grant safety guidelines. We observed that after every house initially voted to allow alcohol consumption, all but one subsequently voted to become dry. This suggests that the model was actually working: clients had learned something valuable about making group decisions among themselves in their best interests rather than having rules imposed from without. However, as a result of this tactic, the grant began to accrue a reputation among some local clinical circles for fostering alcoholism in seriously ill people. This is an example where client empowerment hinges on staff tolerance of decisions which, initially, are apparently "wrong" but lead to higher levels of self-determination.

Similar issues arose over staff control. The staff were told, "You work for the clients. You are to do what they ask you to do as long as it's not dangerous nor dramatically counter-therapeutic." Some staff members initially had laissez-faire attitudes toward empowerment: do nothing, give no advice or information. With more experience, the staff gradually learned that fostering client independence involved some middle ground between being a controlling agent and abandoning responsibility and input.

Lessons for Clinical Research Involving Housing

We have learned that conducting a research project, which requires random selection and assignments, has its costs. Pressures created by that process caused significant difficulties. Specifically, our design prohibited any control over who was assigned to which housing type. In retrospect, we feel that careful matching of housemates within ECHs, and the employment of clinical criteria such as diagnosis, previous substance use, recency of psychiatric hospitalizations, level of functioning, may have led to more "successful" placements within housing types.

Placement into housing took place as units and group homes became available over a period of 18 months. We tried to make the initiation process as uniform as possible across the seven ECH sites. Some natural contamination in the design did occur when, for example, residents of the first ECH volunteered to help the the next ECH group to settle into their new home.

The Boston McKinney project also enlisted two different vendors to manage the various ECHs. This led to differences in management philosophy and style between the ECHs, despite our efforts to instill a uniform empowerment philosophy within the staff of each vendor organization. We would recommend that, should others attempt to replicate the Evolving Consumer Household model, they seriously consider beginning with a single vendor with overall responsibility for multiple project sites so that a consistent policy can be established and maintained.

Project Management Issues

The Achilles heel of the ECH model was the lack of reasonable incentives for staff to work themselves out of their own employment and administrative structures that would facilitate staff transfer. By successfully instilling the empowerment philosophy within the residents and teaching them to be self-reliant, staff rendered themselves superfluous and potentially unemployed. (Vendors in charge of staffing guaranteed each staff member an additional three months of employment elsewhere in their systems). Furthermore, the amount of paperwork for remaining staff increased since licensing and regulatory requirements did not "down-size" over time.

A related implementation problem was our initial notion that clients would lay staff off when they felt they no longer needed them. This proved to be more difficult to implement than we had imagined. The clients, having experienced poverty, found it impossible to lay off anyone. Clients felt that terminating employment was always unreasonable and would wish it on no one. Their solution was to request that individual staff members remain in the staff room within the ECH for the duration of their shifts, thereby maintaining their paycheck while ostensibly removing them from the residents' living space – a "humanitarian" but fiscally unsound practice! Later, we realized that we had not adequately informed the tenants in the houses that reducing staffing in their home would not cost staff their jobs. Rather, it should be made explicit that such staff will be transferred to other programs or used to bring their experience to other similar projects.

The problems connected with planned obsolescence of the staff could be obviated by planning a series of ECH units to be opened over a longer-term period (perhaps five years). If the homes were opened in a deliberately slow sequence, selected staff from the first home could serve as the initiators of the second home, temporarily leaving behind some core "empowerment training" staff at the first home. As the second home develops, the "empowerment team" from the first home would move on to the second home, while the "advance team" would move on to initiate the third home. This would serve several purposes simultaneously: it would foster specialization within the staffing (advance teams vs. empowerment teams), assure longer-term employment for staff, create an atmosphere for learning from earlier homes and applying the experience and knowledge gained to the newer homes, and offer employment opportunities for "graduates" of the homes to serve as peer counselors for newer participants. It is also important to have the option of reinstating staff if the ECH realizes it is not ready for full independence after a reasonable trial period.

We recommend that a more purposeful selection of clients for participation in the ECH model be implemented. Considerations should be given to medication compliance, histories of substance abuse, and past relationships among the participant pool to build on existing friendships. We would also recommend assuring participants that they could opt to relocate to other houses within the system if they feel uncomfortable within the ECH to which they were originally assigned. Since each residence develops its own character, the ability to relocate within the system (subject to the approval of the other residents, of course) would be a highly desirable feature.

We have also recognized that there is a need for respite beds for residents who occasionally need time away from the ECH or their own apartment. Our subjects sometimes filled that need by "eloping" from their assignments from time to time when the situation became unbearable, and returning later when things felt more manageable.

CONCLUSIONS

We feel that we have convincingly demonstrated that when appropriately structured interventions are offered, an extremely high proportion of homeless individuals with severe mental illness, including those who abuse substances, can be engaged effectively and placed into stable housing situations. Only 19% of those individuals who were recruited and placed into housing had returned to living in shelters or on the street by the end of the 18 month follow-up period.

Second, housing that is safe, affordable and acceptable can be developed despite the many bureaucratic obstacles that were encountered in the implementation of this project. Effective housing development requires collaborative relationships among mental health providers, housing agencies, shelter staff and clinicians. Seeking the advice of consumers proved to be a key element in maximizing the acceptability and effectiveness of this project's housing efforts.

Third, consumers are willing to accept both individual housing and group living situations, despite their initial resistance to group living, provided the system is responsive to their needs and willing to incorporate their ideas.

Finally, we have demonstrated that even severely impaired individuals can develop the ability to work together and acquire the skills necessary to handle most of the tasks generally performed by residential staff. The process can be slow and sometimes painful, but with patience and persistence, a large degree of client empowerment is possible.

REFERENCES

Allard, M.A. & Carling, P.J. (1986). *Providing housing and supports for people with psychiatric disabilities*. Washington, DC: NIMH.

Axelroad, S.E. & Toff, G.E. (1987). *Outreach services for homeless ill people*. Washington, DC: The Intergovernmental Health Policy Project, George Washington University.

Barrow, S.M., Hellman, F., Lovell, A.M., Plapinger, J.D. & Struening, E.L. (1989). *Effectiveness of programs for the mentally ill homeless: Final report*. New York: Community Support Systems Evaluation Program, New York State Psychiatric Institute.

Bassuk, E.L. & Lamb, H.R. (1986). Homelessness and the implementation of deinstitutionalization. *New Directions for Mental Health Services* 30:7–14.

Blanch, A.K. & Carling, P.J. (1988). Normal housing with special supports. *Rehabilitation Psychology* 33:47–55.

Carling, P.J. (1990). Major mental illness, housing, and supports: The promise of community integration. *American Psychologist* 45:969–975.

Center for Mental Health Services. (1994). *Making A Difference: Interim Status Report of the McKinney Demonstration Program for Homeless Adults with Serious Mental Illness*. Washington, DC: U.S. Department of Health and Human Services.

Chafetz, L. & Goldfinger, S.M. (1984). Residential instability in a psychiatric emergency setting. *Psychiatric Quarterly* 56:20–34.

Depp, F., Scarpelli, A.E. & Apostoles, F.E. (1983). Making cooperative living work for psychiatric outpatients. *Health and Social Work* 8:271–282.

Elliott, S.J., S.M. Taylor & Kearns, R.A. (1990). Housing satisfaction, preference and need among the chronically mentally disabled in Hamilton, Ontario. *Social Science and Medicine* 30(1):95–102.

Fischer, P.J. & Breakey, W.R. (1986). Homelessness and mental health: An overview. *International Journal of Mental Health*, 14:6–41.

Frances, A.J. & Goldfinger, S.M. (1986). "Treating" a homeless mentally ill patient who cannot be managed in the shelter system. *Hospital and Community Psychiatry* 37:577–579.

Goering, P., Paduchak, D. & Durbin, J. (1990). Housing homeless women: a consumer preference study. *Hospital and Community Psychiatry* 41:790–794.

Goldfinger, S.M., Dickey, B., Good B., Hellman, S., O'Bryan, M., Penk, W.E., Schutt, R.K., Seidman, L.J. & Ware, N. (1990). *Independent Apartments vs. Evolving Consumer Households for Homeless Seriously Mentally Ill Individuals*. Proposal to the National Institute of Mental Health. Funded proposal.

Harris, M. & Bachrach L.L. (Eds.). (1988). *Clinical Case Management*. San Francisco, CA: Jossey Bass.

Harris, M. & Bergman, H.C. (1987). Case management with the chronically mentally ill: A clinical perspective. *American Journal of Orthopsychiatry* 57:296.

Kanter, J.S. (1985). *Clinical Issues in Treating the Chronically Mentally Ill*. San Francisco, CA: Jossey Bass.

Lamb, H.R. (1984). Deinstitutionalization and the homeless mentally ill. *Hospital and Community Psychiatry* 35:899–907.

Levine, I.S. & Parrish, J. (1986). Comments on residential facilities for the mentally ill: Needs assessment and community planning. *Community Mental Health Journal* 22:90–93.

Lipton, F.R., Nutt, S. & Sabatini, A. (1988). Housing the homeless mentally ill: A longitudinal study of a treatment approach. *Hospital and Community Psychiatry* 39:40–45.

Mulkern, V. & Bradley, V.J. (1986). Service utilization and service preferences of homeless persons. *Psychosocial Rehabilitation Journal* 10:23–29.

Ridgway, P., (Ed.), Carling, P.J., Chamberlin, J., Crafts, J., DiPasquale, S., Finkle, M., Harp, H., Hendricks, H., Posey, T., Somerville, F. & Van Tosh, L. (1988). *Coming Home: Ex-Patients View Housing Options and Needs*. Procdings of a National Housing Forum: Boston, MA, 1–34.

Rosen, A., Hadzi-Pavlovic, D. & Parker, G. (1989). The Life Skills Profile: A Measure Assessing Function and Disability in Schizophrenia. *Schizophrenia Bulletin* 15(2):325–337.

Rosenheck, R., Leda, C., Gallup, P. & Astrachan, B.M. (1989). Initial assessment data from a 43-site program for homeless chronic mentally ill veterans. *Hospital and Community Psychiatry* 40:937–942.

Schutt, R.K., Goldfinger, S.M. (in press) Homeless mentally ill persons' residential preferences: the role of health and functioning. *Psychiatric Services*.

Susser, E., Goldfinger, S.M. & White, A. (1990). Some clinical approaches to the homeless mentally ill. Special Issue: The homeless mentally ill. *Community Mental Health Journal* 26:463–480.

Tessler, R.C. & Dennis, D.L. (1989). *A Synthesis of NIMH-Funded Research Concerning Persons Who are Homeless and Mentally Ill*. Washington, DC: NIMH.

Thomas, J.E. (1987). A Study of Expatients' Perspectives on Their Housing Experiences and Options. *Smith College Studies in Social Work* 57(3):199–217.

Ware, J.E. & Sherbourne, C.D. (1992). The MOS 36-Item Short-Form Health Survey (SF-36): Conceptual Framework and Item Selection. *Medical Care* 30(June): 473–483.

NOTE

Research funded by NIMH Grant #1R18MH4808001, Stephen M. Goldfinger, MD, Principal Investigator.

4

Assertive Community Treatment for Homeless Adults with Severe Mental Illness in Baltimore

LISA DIXON, EIMER KERNAN, NANCY KRAUSS, ANTHONY LEHMAN and BRUCE R. DEFORGE

In search of a more effective way to aid persons with severe and persistent mental illnesses who cycled frequently between the hospital and the community, clinician-researchers in Madison, Wisconsin developed the Training in Community Living Program more than two decades ago. This program evolved into the Program for Assertive Community Treatment (PACT) (Stein & Test, 1975; Stein & Test, 1980; Test, 1979). Systematic evaluation has revealed the capacity of PACT to decrease hospitalization and enhance clinical and social outcomes at costs comparable to more traditional service delivery patterns (Weisbrod, Test & Stein, 1980; Olfson, 1990; Burns & Santos, 1995). Building upon this model, the project described here adapted the PACT approach to serve homeless persons with severe and persistent mental illnesses. The goal was to improve the capacity of the service system to serve a target population that was not adequately cared for by the existing array of services.

The original PACT model was developed for persons with mental illness who were destined for hospitalization and had some level of family or community support. During the past decade, others have modified PACT principles and applied them in different settings including inner-city and rural environments and to other client groups, including dual diagnosis clients and outpatients with high levels of service utilization (Olfson, 1990; Burns & Santos, 1995; Essock & Kontos, 1995; Teague, Drake & Ackerson, 1995). In this

51

project, we applied PACT to yet another group, homeless persons with severe mental illnesses. In order to evaluate the effectiveness of the PACT model in a homeless population, homeless persons with mental illnesses who were recruited for the project were randomized to the new experimental condition, The Assertive Community Treatment (ACT) team (modeled on the PACT approach), or to the control condition which consisted of the usual and customary mental health and social services available in Baltimore City.

The project represented the coordinated efforts of a community mental health center (the Walter P. Carter Center), a university research program (Center for Mental Health Services Research at the University of Maryland), a provider of health services for the homeless (Health Care for the Homeless), and a homeless shelter (Project PLASE), all under the organizing sponsorship of a city-wide local mental health authority (Baltimore Mental Health Systems, Inc). In addition, four co-investigators represented departments of anthropology, mental hygiene, social work, and community psychiatry.

EXPERIMENTAL INTERVENTION: THE ASSERTIVE COMMUNITY TREATMENT (ACT) TEAM

Mission and Philosophy

The mission of the ACT team is to provide comprehensive services to homeless persons with severe mental illnesses in Baltimore City who have been unable to make use of traditional outpatient mental health services. The package of services includes direct clinical case management, medical and psychiatric care, social work services, as well as some housing options. The team philosophy is that by engaging individuals in a non-threatening and non-intrusive way, assisting them to secure housing, entitlements, psychiatric and medical care, and helping them to function in the community, their quality of life will improve. This can only be achieved if the autonomy and preferences of individuals are respected.

Staffing and Roles

The team is composed of professionals and consumers; Figure 4.1 describes its organizational structure. In addition to the permanent staff, the program has attracted two half-time senior psychiatric residents per year: ten residents have worked with the program to date. Two social work students and one nursing student have also trained with the program.

The Clinical Director is responsible for program administration including program development, personnel issues, securing on-going program funds and overseeing day-to-day operations. The Medical Director has overall clinical responsibility for the psychiatric care delivered by the team. In addition, the Medical Director carries a caseload of 15–20 clients and supervises psychiatric resi-

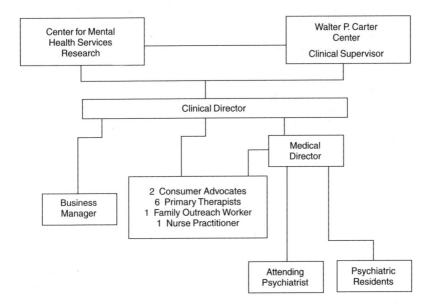

Figure 4.1. Clinical team components.

dents. A staff psychiatrist has a caseload of 15–20 clients. Psychiatric residents have primary responsibility for a caseload of 12–15 clients and work with the Medical Director to provide psychiatric services, education, and consultation to the rest of the team.

Nurses, social workers, and counselors act as clinical case managers (CCM). CCMs are primary therapists and carry their own caseloads. Although staff did not act as primary therapists for specific patients in the original PACT model, we found that the long engagement phase and the isolation these homeless people had experienced necessitated that we assign a primary therapist to each individual to enable the formation of a therapeutic relationship. The CCMs provide direct service and make referrals to outside agencies when appropriate (e.g., intensive substance abuse treatment or vocational rehabilitation). CCMs have a relatively low caseload (10–12 patients), allowing them to provide supportive counseling, psychoeducation, help with money management, and assistance in obtaining entitlements, clothing, shelter, medical care, and housing. The CCM is the "point person" and the conduit of information, developing treatment plans in conjunction with the clients and the rest of the treatment team. The CCMs try to make sure that their clients get the services they need. CCMs who are nurses assess medical needs, are responsible for administering medication injections, and keep the medication records in order.

The two full-time consumer advocates have histories of mental illness and/or homelessness. Consumer advocates act as bridges

Table 4.1. Assertive Community Treatment (ACT) Clients Demographics (N = 77)

	N	%	
Gender			
Male	50	64.9	
Female	27	35.1	
Race			
White (non-hispanic)	27	35.1	
African American	47	61.0	
Hispanic	2	2.6	
Other	1	1.3	
Age			
< 26 yrs	7	9.1	
26-35 yrs	25	32.5	
36-45 yrs	32	41.6	
> 45 yrs	13	16.9	(Mean age 38.6 ± 9.5)
Education			
<HS graduate	41	54.7	
HS graduate	23	30.7	
College plus	11	14.7	(Mean grade 10.8 ± 2.9)
Marital status			
Ever married	32	42.1	
Never married	44	57.9	
Armed Forces-veteran			
Yes	15	19.5	
Time spent homeless[1]			
Less than 3 months	4	8.2	
3-11 months	8	16.3	
1-3 years	18	36.7	
4-9 years	13	26.5	
10 years or more	6	12.2	
Years in Baltimore			
< 1 year	6	8.0	
1-5 years	15	20.0	
6-10 years	5	6.7	
16-20 years	4	5.3	
>20 years	45	60.0	

Table 4.1. Continued

	N	%
DSM-III-R **Principal Axis I Diagnosis** **(SCID)^2**		
Bipolar disorder	13	16.9
Major depression	4	5.2
NOS depressive disorder	1	1.3
Schizophrenia	35	45.5
Schizoaffective	11	14.3
NOS psychotic disorder	1	1.3
Alcohol	8	10.4
Cocaine	3	3.9
Generalized anxiety	1	1.3
Substance abuse/dependence **(SCID)^2**		
Yes	55	71.4

[1]28 individuals were unable to give a specific time frame.
[2]SCID = Structured Clinical Interview for DSM-III-R.

between the treatment team and the clients, providing the perspective of someone who has "been there." They provide peer counseling, client advocacy, and education for clients as well as staff. This will be discussed in more detail later in the chapter. The family outreach worker works with the ACT team by contract with the Alliance for the Mentally Ill of Maryland. She contacts family members for support and education, and often has family meetings with the staff and clients.

The nurse practitioner provides services to all clients of the ACT team. She is responsible for conducting physical examinations, assessing clients' medical needs, providing direct treatment for chronic medical problems, and coordinating medical care with other appropriate agencies.

Description of Clients

The major characteristics of the 77 ACT clients are presented in Table 4.1. Approximately two-thirds are male, with an average age of 38.6 years (±9.5 years). Just over 60 percent are African American, while slightly over one-third are white. At the time of referral to the program, 60 percent of the clients reported that they lived in Baltimore for over 20 years, while relatively few, (8 percent) had resided in the city for less than a year. Nearly one-half had been homeless for 1 year or more; 36 percent of the clients could not determine the amount of time they had spent homeless. Prior to their entry into the ACT program, over one-third of the clients reported they had lived on the streets (37 percent) or in a group home or a shelter (37 percent) while only a handful (9 percent) were staying in a house or apartment. About 17 percent of the ACT clients were hospitalized at the time of referral.

Nearly 46 percent of the ACT clients have schizophrenia, 14 percent have schizoaffective disorder while almost a quarter have a major affective disorder. Only 14 percent of the clients have a substance use disorder as their primary diagnosis, although over 70 percent meet the DSM-III-R criteria for co-occurring psychoactive substance use disorders.

Working with Clients

Each person referred to the ACT team is assigned to a "mini-team" composed of a CCM, a psychiatrist and a consumer advocate. However, the entire team works together in decision making and each staff member is knowledgeable about most of the clients. This team work is fostered through twice weekly team meetings in which treatment plans are developed and through daily "signout" meetings in which the work of each day is reviewed and the next day's work is reported and planned. On several occasions, clients have switched primary case managers or doctors when this is clinically indicated. This process has been facilitated by the team's shared knowledge of all clients.

ACT staff members are accessible 24 hours a day. The office is open from 8:30 A.M. to 5 P.M., Monday through Friday. When the office is closed, an on-call ACT therapist carries a beeper. The on-call therapist is expected to be available for crisis intervention counseling by telephone. The Clinical Program Director and a psychiatrist are available for back-up at all times. All clients are given a laminated card identifying them as part of the ACT team. Our emergency telephone number appears on the card.

We have organized the experience of working with our clients into four phases:

1) Engagement;

2) Stabilization;

3) Ongoing Treatment and Maintenance; and

4) Discharge.

Not all of the individuals referred to the program pass through each of these phases, nor are these phases necessarily always connected in a linear fashion. Nevertheless, this framework has helped us to conceptualize where individuals stand with respect to their work with the program. An additional component of the services ACT employs is tracking clients who leave treatment. The tracking component can operate in any of the phases, but typically is most important during the engagement phase.

Engagement: The goal of the engagement phase is to develop a trusting relationship between the treatment team and the client. Engagement is successful when clients identify the team as their service provider. Many homeless people with severe mental illness have had negative experiences with established agencies and care providers. The ACT team interacts with referred individuals in many ways to achieve this trust. An essential ingredient of this process is determining what the individual wants. The team helps clients meet basic needs and provides material support such as meals, bus tokens, laundry money and perhaps most important, shelter. The team goes into the community and spends time simply talking and getting to know the person. Treatment and medication may be offered, but not required. The team often follows clients through psychiatric hospitalizations, episodes of substance use, arrests, and disappearances to let them know that we will be persistent and supportive. For some, this phase takes an entire year. Others engage quickly, particularly if they have a specific need that ACT can help them to meet, such as housing or psychiatric care.

The following case example illustrates the engagement process for one client:

Ms. S is a 32-year-old divorced white woman with a diagnosis of schizophrenia and substance abuse, referred to the team by a drop-in center. At the time of referral she was not taking medication on a regular basis and had been drinking alcohol heavily. The team went to the center to meet Ms S where her chief complaint was needing a place to stay for the night and a pack of cigarettes. The team located a bed for Ms. S at the transitional shelter used by ACT. She left the shelter shortly after arriving that night, apparently sleeping on the streets. The next night, the team found a bed at a different shelter. Through the next week Ms S became disruptive at that shelter and was asked to leave. Our contact with Ms S then became sporadic. We made many attempts to contact Ms S, leaving letters and messages at the drop-in center and other facilities she frequented. Three months after referral, we received a call from the drop-in center: Ms S was there and exhibiting bizarre behavior. The team psychiatrist, consumer advocate and therapist went to see Ms S. By the time all arrived, Ms S had left the center and was headed down the street.

The three team members drove around the streets and caught up with Ms S. She was agitated, thought disordered, and appeared jaundiced, an indication of liver disease. An Emergency Petition was filed. The police brought Ms S to an emergency room. She was admitted to the hospital and stayed for two weeks. After her discharge we again lost contact with Ms S for 3 weeks. We learned that she was living with her boyfriend who assisted us in helping Ms S. We also applied to become the representative payee for Ms S's Social Security check to assure that she had funds to pay for a place to stay. We had learned that she had previously arranged to have her check deposited directly to the account of a local liquor store. It was not until another 3 months had elapsed and another hospitalization that Ms S came into our office stating that she would like to work with the ACT team. We assisted her in finding a room to rent and became her representative payee. While her contacts with the team were crisis oriented, she slowly became more engaged with the team. She began coming to the office several times a week. Ms S now has a Section 8 apartment which she shares with her boyfriend. ACT pays her rent and utilities with her check, and she gets an allowance twice a week. She has obtained furniture, is taking medication and is relatively stable. She still comes in crisis and calls when she is distressed, but we also see her when she is not in crisis.

Stabilization: During this phase, clients begin to develop skills necessary to maintain themselves in stable community housing. Long-term housing, income, daily structure, chronic medical problems, substance abuse, family and relationship issues, and psychiatric care are addressed. Generally, each client is willing or interested in working on some, if not all, of these issues. Critical to the identification of goals is the active participation of clients in the process. We have found that if preferences and desires of clients are not integral to the development of goals, these clients leave treatment. Strategies used in this phase are discussed in more detail below.

Ongoing treatment and maintenance: The goal of this phase is to help clients maintain the gains and progress they have made. The lifestyles and circumstances of our clients often change dramatically over a year or two; people who have lived on the streets for 20 years now have an independent apartment. We have found that maintaining stability is itself a goal, even though it may appear that the client is not moving forward. Clients in this phase often require a lower intensity of services, but are not yet ready for discharge from ACT.

Mr. C was referred to the ACT team from a local homeless provider agency. He had been living on the streets for 10 years, had a history of alcoholism, and a diagnosis of schizophrenia and many somatic problems. He was receiving public assistance and food stamps and panhandled for extra funds. The ACT team referred Mr. C for treatment for his more severe medical problems, applied and obtained social security benefits, and became his representative payee. He obtained a Section 8 apartment and began regularly coming to the ACT team for medication and money. Mr C has been with the ACT team for three years. He currently maintains himself in housing. During the day he frequents his old stomping ground and comes to the ACT office to attend our dual diagnosis groups. He is compliant with medication and keeps all of his medical appointments. While he continues to have alcoholic binges every month or so, he is otherwise psychiatrically stable.

Discharge: All ACT clients are reviewed annually for appropriateness of continuing in the ACT program. Discharge can be considered when one of the following occurs:

1) the goals and objectives of the treatment plan are met and the client can be transferred to a less intensive mental health care program;

2) the client proves not to have an Axis I psychiatric diagnosis;

3) the client's only Axis I diagnosis is a substance abuse or dependence disorder;

4) the client is institutionalized in another treatment or correctional facility and it is expected that the client will remain there for a period greater than 3 months;

5) the client moves out of the Baltimore area;

6) the client dies;

7) the client has not actively engaged in treatment with the ACT team for a 3-month period and all efforts to re-engage the client have failed.

In practice, the majority of our discharges have occurred when clients have been lost to follow-up. A few clients have actively chosen to leave the team, and a few have been discharged and referred because they have substance disorders only.

Discharge to a less intensive mental health program has proven to be as difficult as engagement; the difficulty in discharge is probably related to the difficulty in engagement. Having established what is for many clients the first positive relationship with service providers, it is difficult to terminate that relationship, especially within only one or two years. Further, many clients appear to need an intensity of services which is greater than what is typically available in standard programs. The following case is an example of one client in the process of a planned discharge.

Ms J and the ACT team are working towards discharge to a more traditional mental health service. Ms J carries a diagnosis of major depression and personality disorder with dependent features. During the course of her work with the ACT team, she has maintained herself in the community in a Section 8 apartment, attended training to learn computer skills and is currently in individual psychotherapy at a mental health clinic. Our first attempt to move Ms J towards discharge was met with difficulty. She began to decompensate. We supported her and continued our treatment with her. After a period, she felt more comfortable with her therapist at the mental health clinic. In addition, she is being referred to a case management program in her area. They will continue to follow Ms J and make sure that she is doing well in the community. Our plan is to phase out our treatment with Ms J over.the next six months.

Tracking: The tracking component of the program mobilizes when we cannot locate a client. The consumer advocates who have been homeless provide much guidance with tracking. As early as possible in the relationship, staff try to get an idea of where on the streets clients spend their time. Advocates are familiar with the city shelters, soup kitchens and other areas where homeless people spend time. If a patient whom we generally see on a daily basis suddenly stops coming to the clinic, the advocate and usually the client's primary therapist make telephone calls and search the streets for this person. If the person stays at a local shelter, we will try to determine when the client was last seen there. If this fails, we begin to call local hospitals, the jail, and the morgue. The team always seeks consent from new clients to speak with other service providers should the need arise.

> Mr. T is a 30 year old man with a diagnosis of schizophrenia who was referred to the ACT team while hospitalized. During the course of early conversations with Mr. T, the team learned of his habit of going to peep shows. Prior to Mr T's discharge, he eloped from the hospital. The team was notified and did some tracking on the streets to find Mr T. After much searching on foot, the team found Mr T at a peep show. He said that he did not return for fear that the team would be angry with him. When he found that the team was not angry and located space for him at a shelter, he continued his work with ACT. There have been other occasions when Mr T has been missing from the Baltimore area and was located out-of-state through networking (mostly with his mother) and the fact that he had an ACT ID card.

Problem Areas and Interventions

Mental illness: The majority of ACT clients suffer from severe and persistent psychiatric disorders. Interventions start at the time of the engagement phase with a focus on building trust between the client and the team. We use psychotropic medications, psycho-education, hospitalization, and psychotherapy with behavioral, cognitive and psychological approaches. In general, we try to find the right balance of flexibility and structure. Strategies to enhance medication compliance include individual packaging of medication dosages and close supervision of medication by ACT staff or other providers in the community. Clients are carefully evaluated for past histories of side-effects. The ACT team can provide direct inpatient care at a local state hospital and community mental health facility. If clients refuse medication or if we are concerned that approaching them about medication may interfere with the engagement process, clients are still followed and seen regularly by psychiatrists. The idea is that we will "walk with the clients" where they need to go, and be there to persuade, to clarify, and to provide emergency services. Psychiatric staff initiate emergency petitions if clients are in acute danger. A small supply of stock medications are available in the ACT office if medication is required urgently. Emergencies are referred to the University Hospital Emergency Room.

Homelessness: As all of the clients who are referred to the ACT team are homeless, many for more than 5 years, the team immediately develops a short-term and long-term housing plan. This plan is developed in conjunction with the clients, balancing their wants and needs, their clinical status, and available resources. Short-term housing options include motel (often paid for by ACT client assistance funds), psychiatric or medical hospitalization (if necessary), residential crisis beds, family, and transitional shelter beds or missions. The program has access to supervised transitional shelter beds (10 the first year, 8 the second year, and 6 the third year). There is generally a waiting list for these beds. Few clients have income or available money at the time of referral, so options are limited.

Long-term housing plans are made after engagement is successful. Long-term housing options include board and care homes, single room occupancy dwellings and independent apartments, including Section 8 housing (Section 8 housing is a Federally funded, locally administered rental assistance program for low income individuals and families. Under the program, recipients pay 30% of their income to rent and utilities; the local Housing Authority pays the remainder directly to the landlord). The decision about which option to pursue is developed collaboratively with the client as part of the treatment plan. The team works with the client in an attempt to prepare and support the client in whatever housing option the client wishes. For example, if the client is pursuing independent living in an apartment, staff will work with the client on the skills of independent living such as shopping, keeping an apartment clean, and budgeting.

Sometimes clients do not wish to pursue stable housing. In this case, the team tries not to impose its values or wishes upon the client. The team will work with the client in whatever ways we agree we can help, and will keep reviewing the client's choice. Often, the client will eventually change his or her mind. Sometimes the team and the client disagree about what the client can safely handle. These situations are negotiated on an individual basis. Generally, the team will support what the client wants, except if the team feels that the clients' choice constitutes a severe risk to their health.

Clients with substance abuse problems and mental illness pose other problems related to housing. Many shelters will not accept clients who are dually diagnosed or are currently using substances. Shelters which accept people with addiction histories often have strict rules. Clients may be required to attend Alcoholics or Narcotics Anonymous meetings or submit to urine screens. Clients may not wish to do this, especially if they do not feel that they have a substance abuse problem. In these cases, we do our best to determine what we think is the most therapeutic for the client. Some clients are motivated by rules and need firm limits. However, others will continue to flounder on the streets if they are only given housing options which have a requirement of abstinence. We have found that there is a fine line between "enabling" substance abuse and providing a suitable environment with housing in which clients can begin to struggle with their addiction.

Money and income: Many ACT clients either have no income at the time of referral or have been unable to manage their income to provide for their basic needs. The team makes an immediate assessment of clients' entitlements and, if appropriate, will either initiate or continue the process of obtaining benefits. Most of our clients are disabled and qualify for Supplemental Security Income (SSI) or Social Security Disability Income (SSDI). However, many have been unable to negotiate the process of applying for SSI/SSDI or have not been in one place long enough to complete an application. If a client already receives an income, the team will assess the need for a representative payee and will be the representative payee, if necessary. The use of a representative payee is particularly appropriate for those using drugs or alcohol.

As the representative payee, the team makes a budget with the client and will pay rent, utility bills, and purchase food and clothing. Allowances are given to some on a daily basis, and others on a weekly or monthly basis. Clients who abuse substances will often not receive any cash; their therapist or consumer advocate will go grocery shopping with them and purchase all of their needed items.

The practice of the therapist handling the funds (setting up the budget with the client and actually giving the client money) has at times interfered with the therapeutic relationship. It is often difficult to get beyond money issues. In these cases, another person may be assigned to negotiate money, and the therapist can maintain a therapeutic relationship. The ultimate goal is for all clients to be able to manage their funds effectively and independently.

Funds are kept in a separate representative payee account at a local bank. Clients' checks are deposited directly into that account. On a weekly basis, therapists request funds needed for the following week. Requests are submitted to the Program Director who obtains money from the bank and keeps track of the accounting for these funds. Large purchases are paid for by check. While we try to avoid power struggles around money and to give clients as much control as possible, the team will not avoid stepping in to help provide control if the client clearly cannot meet his/her basic needs without help.

Medical illness: Acute and chronic medical problems are common among homeless people. The team nurse practitioner provides direct medical care. The office has an examining room equipped with an examining table and other basic medical equipment. The nurse practitioner evaluates all clients taking a medical history and conducting a physical exam. She initiates and maintains treatment for non-acute medical problems (diabetes, hypertension, routine infections, etc.), provides medical teaching, routine foot care, and coordinates the client's medical care when it is necessary to use outside physicians or services. The ACT team and the nurse practitioner have an arrangement for consultations with the Family Practice Clinic at the University of Maryland. ACT attempts to encourage clients to centralize care for all their medical problems and not use the emergency room. Of note, it was difficult to find a nurse practitioner willing and qualified to work with this population.

Activities of daily living: rehabilitation: Many ACT clients lack skills in basic areas such as shopping, budgeting and hygiene. For some, simply being provided with the resources, such as money or a shower, solves the problem. However, others need more assistance. ACT team staff accompany clients to shop for clothes, furniture, food and the like, and help with budgeting and paying bills. Additionally, ACT staff work with clients on personal hygiene. If clients lack skills in basic arithmetic and reading, we refer them to literacy and educational programs. Staff make home visits where necessary to help achieve these goals.

Rehabilitation in this context means helping individuals to regain (or gain for the first time) the living skills they need to function in the community, as well as to achieve vocational and social goals. The tasks of rehabilitation generally do not become relevant until the individual has engaged with and trusts the team, when their basic needs have been met, and the client and the team can turn their attention to the future. The ACT program utilizes several community programs to help with rehabilitation, as well as providing some activities within the program itself. For example, ACT staff will go shopping, work on budgeting (see money section), and participate in recreational activities with clients. This is especially important for those clients who have difficulty engaging with any other treatment system. The program also uses Harbor City Unlimited (HCU), a psychosocial rehabilitation program. The ACT team and HCU are housed in the same building, so it is very convenient for ACT clients to "go upstairs to HCU". This program has training opportunities in secretarial, custodial, and cooking skills and is very flexibly structured. It seems to work best for clients who need a low-demand, low-structure setting. Clients are also referred to other programs in Baltimore City that provide vocational rehabilitation and job skills training.

Family: A high proportion of ACT clients have little or no family contact at referral. Anger, guilt and grief characterize the feelings clients express when talking about their families. The ACT team encourages clients on an individual basis to enhance their family relationships. The family outreach consultant, a family member with two immediate relatives who have mental illness, has proven to be a unique and valuable member of the team. The consultant participates in the intake and treatment planning process, helping the team to understand the family perspective. The family consultant attempts to gain the trust of clients so they will give their permission to contact their families. She has helped families to increase their understanding of the client's illness, behavior, and the need for, and the side effects of, medication. She has initiated written correspondence with family members who have no phone or live far away. She has taken day trips of several hundred miles with clients and their therapist to make a home visit.

Substance abuse: Substance addiction is common among ACT clients. Before any substance abuse treatment intervention can be developed, the client must be engaged with treatment and trust the team. This means that the team does not address the substance abuse immediately, unless it is a medical emergency. We have adopted a model for treatment of people with dual diagnoses advanced by Osher and Kofoed (1989) which defines four phases: engagement; persuasion; active treatment; and relapse prevention. We try to persuade clients to enter treatment by pointing out, repetitively if necessary, how their addiction is causing them problems. Their homelessness is often powerful evidence of the consequences of addiction. The team has a dual diagnosis treatment group which meets three times a week for one hour. We encourage the use of AA and NA where appropriate and have had staff members attend meetings with clients. We also utilize psychiatric hospitalization, detoxification and 28-day rehabilitation programs. In addition, the team consults with an addiction psychiatrist every other week. The focus of the consultation is to develop creative treatment plans with clients who do not accept conventional addiction treatment options. Integrating treatment for substance abuse with money management, medical and psychiatric care, and housing is critical. Philosophically, we do not give ultimatums or require substance abuse treatment as a condition of further ACT care. We will, however, work with the legal system or Probation Officer if clients have developed legal problems as a result of their substance abuse. Substance abuse is a challenging problem in this population because it is difficult, on the one hand, for people to address their substance abuse while they are coping with the problem of homelessness. On the other hand, substance abuse often leads to loss of housing. We have had to locate housing options in the community where some substance abuse is tolerated as long as clients do not present a danger to themselves or others in the home. We have also found that as long as we pay the rent through the representative payee mechanism, clients who abuse drugs and alcohol can often maintain their housing even in the presence of ongoing use. Another useful strategy has been advocating with housing providers to be more flexible in dealing with the substance abuse problems of our clients.

Daily structure: Some clients attend day treatment or psychosocial programs, job training or employment. Others have non-traditional ways of structuring their time such as going to peepshows, walking the streets, window shopping or just coming into the ACT office. We have learned not to push daily structure to meet our needs, but to listen to clients and assist them when necessary.

Special Resources

Client assistance: Discretionary funds are available through the grant for client use. Staff typically purchase bus tokens, food, clothing, emergency shelter such as motel beds, and personal items for clients. Most funds are spent during the engagement process when clients have no income. A significant portion of client assistance funds are devoted to purchasing medications for clients who have no insurance.

Housing: The research project acquired forty Section 8 certificates which were available to clients in both the experimental treatment group and the control condition. These were awarded on a first-come first-served basis. In order for clients to apply for a Section 8 certificate through the ACT team, the client must be able to live safely in an independent apartment. To obtain a certificate, clients go through the Section 8 application process which includes two interviews: one at the Baltimore City Housing Authority and one at Baltimore Mental Health Systems Housing Committee. After receiving a certificate the team helps the client to locate an apartment.

The project also utilizes transitional shelter beds at Project PLASE, purchased by the grant and available to clients in both research conditions (Project PLASE is a private, non-profit agency that provides emergency shelter to homeless persons with mental illnesses. Project PLASE is staffed 24 hours per day, provides 3 meals, and supervises medication).

Other issues

Integrating consumers and professionals: The collaboration between consumers and professionals on the team was a unique dimension of the project which we feel has contributed significantly to its success. Without consumers, we probably would have been much less successful in engaging clients and maintaining their participation in services. We are convinced that consumer advocates play an important in role in helping clients to identify and meet their goals. Consumers are instrumental in engaging and tracking clients, providing peer counseling, serving as a role model for clients and professional staff, reducing stigma and educating staff. The consumer advocates often give the team credibility in the eyes of potential clients, and bridge the sometimes vast chasm between clients and staff. Their experiences with medication, addiction, and the psychiatric and homeless service systems provide a wealth of knowledge and sensitivity otherwise unavailable. The participation of consumer advocates undoubtedly enriched the experience of both staff and clients of the ACT Team.

At the same time as the "marriage" of consumers and professionals on a multidisciplinary treatment team provide numerous benefits, this collaboration is also challenging and requires that all individuals involved participate in an ongoing dialogue. Some questions raised by our experience need to be explored and discussed further. These include how to define the role of the consumer advocate, what the boundaries between the consumer advocate and the clients served by the team should be, and how supervision, training and support should be conceptualized and delivered to consumer advocates. The consumer advocate is not a "professional," and may be more effective because of the lack of identification as such. However, it seems that some "professionalization" of consumer advocates needs to occur in order for the team to function effectively. Addressing these challenges is in itself beneficial and in no way detracts from the important roles that consumers have on the team. These issues have been discussed more extensively elsewhere (Dixon, Krauss & Lehman, 1994).

Starting up: The ACT program was started de novo, so every aspect of the program's operation needed to be developed. This included the following structural issues: renovating office space, purchasing equipment and supplies, defining roles and hiring staff, and purchasing cars and insurance. The clinical operation of the program required the development of a schedule for meetings, an infrastructure for documentation and record keeping, a supervisory mechanism, a relationship with a contractual pharmacy for medication, and contracts with other service providers.

After these basic issues were addressed, the most difficult aspect of starting up involved integrating into the community and being accepted by community agencies. We needed to show other agencies that we could work with homeless mentally ill persons and deliver comprehensive services. Regular communication was necessary to avoid conflicts around "ownership of clients," splitting, and to establish trust.

Office location: The ACT team office is located in the community in a storefront building, rather than a hospital or other mental health clinic. It was anticipated that such a location would be conducive to engaging clients who might be reluctant to come to a hospital-like setting, especially if they did not identify themselves as mentally ill or if they had previous negative experience with mental health treatment providers.

Careful thought went into designing the office for safety. It is is located in a high crime and drug area, and money and medication are kept on the premises. We installed metal grates on the windows and an alarm system like other stores. The front door is locked, and the receptionist must buzz people in. A lobby/waiting area with a coffee service is separated from staff offices and meeting rooms by a glass window and walls. The receptionist sits behind the window which is generally kept open. The door leading to staff office space is kept locked and accessible only by a key or buzzer at the reception desk. The Medical Director and Clinical Program Director have separate offices. There is a conference room for groups, case conferences and lunch. Staff share two separate areas for offices which have desks and file cabinets. While this arrangement is problematic for therapists who have private sessions with clients and who need a quiet space to do paperwork, it maximizes team communication and was the best option given the size of the space.

Documentation: The ACT team keeps records in a manner consistent with the rules and regulations for Community Mental Health Centers in the state of Maryland. This includes monthly therapist progress notes, at least quarterly psychiatric notes on medication, and treatment plans with long-term and short-term goals and interventions (outlined within four client contacts and renewed every 90 days thereafter). Records of medication are maintained in a medication order book and psychiatrists must document any medication changes, the rationale for such changes, and that risks and benefits of medications have been explained to clients. Therapists must record the client's progress toward goals outlined in the treatment plans. Clients must be aware of their rights and documentation of this must appear in the chart. Individual charts are reviewed randomly on a monthly basis by the ACT Quality Assurance committee for adherence to these requirements.

Quality assurance; supervision: The quality of the care provided by the ACT team is monitored in three ways. The first is via a formal Quality Assurance (QA) mechanism. On a monthly basis, a staff group consisting of a case manager and psychiatrist or program director review all of the charts of one of the other case managers on the team. Charts are reviewed for all required forms, treatment plans, and appropriate documentation of treatment goals and interventions.

Quality of care is also monitored by the Medical Director and Program Director. The Medical Director meets with all non-psychiatric staff on a biweekly basis and all psychiatric staff weekly. All cases are reviewed in these meetings. The Program Director meets with all staff monthly. Group meetings for treatment planning and "sign out" represent a third QA mechanism. These meetings provide a forum for group supervision and problem solving.

Billing: The ACT team has complied with all regulations necessary to receive a Medicaid number. This allows us to bill for office-based services provided by a mental health professional. We cannot currently bill for services in the community except if clients are living on the streets. We cannot receive reimbursement for services provided to clients in the inpatient setting or for the valuable services provided by the consumer advocate.

Staff morale: Burnout and frustration are ever-present dangers for professionals working with clients who have so many severe problems. Peer support has probably been the most important strategy utilized to minimize burnout. We learned quickly that we need to set modest goals and give positive feedback to each other for jobs well-done. Individual and team meetings are critical for reminding each other of our successes, dealing with our apparent failures, and maintaining boundaries. For staff who are interested, supervision can focus on developing small projects or writing about aspects of the team's work which is a way to balance the sometimes tedious and slow-moving clinical work.

Training: The ACT team has been a training site for senior residents in psychiatry, as well as nursing and social work students. Trainees have added a great deal of excitement and commitment to the program. They help to reduce burnout in the permanent staff. However, having trainees means that clients and permanent staff must adjust to frequent comings and goings which can be very stressful.

THE EVALUATION

Hypotheses

The goal of the research component is to test the following hypotheses:

1) The ACT program increases access to general health and mental health services.

2) The ACT program increases access to basic social services and necessities including stable housing, food, and social entitlements.

3) The ACT program enhances mental health, general health, functional status, and quality of life and reduces family burden.

4) Specific relationships exist between improved access to services and basic necessities and client outcomes. For example, better access to mental health services predicts better mental health outcomes; enhanced access to housing predicts better housing outcomes.

5) The service and outcome effects of the ACT program identified in hypotheses 1–3 differ between those clients who entered from a hospital and those who entered from street and shelter outreach.

6) Total costs under the ACT model are no more than the cost of usual services.

Research Design

Participants in the study were homeless persons with severe and persistent mental illnesses who were recruited from several inpatient sites in Baltimore City and from shelters, soup kitchens, missions, and directly from street locations. Screening and recruitment took place over a nineteen-month period from March, 1991 to September, 1992. Each referral was extensively screened by trained clinicians and included a formal psychiatric diagnostic evaluation. These evaluations took place at all sites that referred clients to the project.

All those eligible for the project had to meet the following criteria:

1) living in Baltimore City for at least 50 percent of the past six months;

2) between 18 and 64 years of age;

3) English speaking, and;

4) legally competent to give consent. Severe and persistent mental illness was defined by diagnosis, duration and disability.

Each person selected had to have a major mental illness in accordance with DSM-III-R criteria as well as a substantial history of psychiatric hospitalizations or persistent functional disability. The definition of homelessness was based on a concept of "literal homelessness" which required one of the following:

1) five days of street or shelter living in the past 45 days or 14 days in the past six months;

2) staying in temporary accommodation (motel room or with a friend or relative) for less than 45 days and at least two moves of accommodation in the past six months.

When clients were determined to be eligible for the study and gave consent, they were randomized on the spot to either the ACT or control conditions. If a client was randomized to ACT, the team was called immediately to arrange a face-to-face meeting. If a client was randomized to the control condition, the referring agency was notified.

Each participant was paid $20 per interview for a total of five interviews which were conducted at baseline (two interviews) and then at two, six, and twelve month follow-up time points. In addition, each participant was asked to name a family member who could be interviewed at baseline and twelve months to assess family burden.

Trained lay and clinical interviewers conducted the research interviews which lasted from sixty to ninety minutes. Areas of assessment included psychiatric diagnosis, service patterns, housing status, mental and general health status, functional status, use of alcohol and drugs, psychiatric symptomatology, and overall life satisfaction. All care providers, both at the ACT team and those treating control group clients, were mailed a Case Manager/Primary Therapist questionnaire at two and twelve months post-referral. This instrument sought information on client need and treatment interventions. A Client Information System (CIS), maintained by the local mental health authority, was used to collect service utilization data for the control group to compare with service/treatment logs completed each week by the ACT team.

Research Issues

Subject recruitment: A total of 1,453 individuals were screened for the project: 183 were eligible, of whom 49 were psychiatric inpatients and 134 were from street and shelter locations. One hundred and fifty two clients (83 percent of those eligible) agreed to participate. Nine of those who were eligible refused (0.6 percent of those eligible), and consent was not obtained from 22 people due to clinical and situational considerations.

The screening figures show that many individuals referred to the project did not meet the eligibility criteria. Overall, 12.5 percent of those screened were eligible; however this rate differed considerably between street and shelter sites and inpatient sites. Of 308 referrals from street and shelter locations, 134 were eligible (43.5 percent); of 1,145 inpatients screened, 49 (4.2 percent) met the eligibility criteria.

As all new inpatient admissions to a downtown community mental health center were screened, it was to be expected that the majority would not meet our homelessness criteria. However, there were fewer individuals available for the project that earlier work had indicated. Most of the street and shelter referrals screened out did not have a severe and persistent mental illness.

The eligibility criteria selected for the study were designed to target persons with severe and persistent mental illness who were "literally homeless". These individuals could be dually diagnosed, but a substance use disorder alone was not sufficient; an additional Axis I disorder was required. When we operationalized the eligibility criteria we found that while we were successful in identifying the target population, we were also screening out many individuals whom community providers thought would benefit from the program. This posed a dilemma for the study: Should we expand the criteria to include more of these individuals, or should we restrict the study to only those individuals who met our specific definition of homelessness and severe mental illness? After careful review of the alternatives we decided not to alter our criteria despite the low eligibility rate. Instead, in order to reach our target number (10 subjects per month over 16 months for the total of 160) we mounted a much more extensive recruitment effort including:

1) expanding the inpatient screening to a second inpatient facility;

2) accepting referrals from other inpatient sites across the city;

3) obtaining permission from three night shelters and two day shelters in the city to conduct on-site psychiatric evaluations;

4) accompanying outreach workers from Heath Care for the Homeless (HCH) on street and shelter outreach;

5) holding bimonthly staff meetings with the mental health team at HCH to review and coordinate referrals; and

6) frequenting locations where homeless persons congregated (e.g., soup kitchens, parks, inner city neighborhoods and the library). In addition, the research team began attending mental health clinics run by HCH staff at several day shelters in the city and meetings of homeless providers held by the Mayor's Office on the Homeless. We also established links with the inpatient discharge planning network operated by the local mental health authority. Although this effort involved a significant investment of time and personnel, it clearly helped the project recruit a suitable sample size.

Subject eligibility: One issue that challenged the research team throughout the screening process was making the correct clinical decision whether an individual met the screening criteria. In particular, the difficulty centered on disentangling substance use disorders from mental illness. It was often extremely difficult to obtain an accurate history and rare to have a relative's collateral history available. Many of the persons referred to the project had experienced severe trauma during childhood, started using substances early in life, received inpatient psychiatric treatment, had family histories positive for mental illness, had not achieved expected milestones, and were currently unemployed in addition to being homeless. Disentangling the sequence of events was very challenging. Moreover, because of the nature of the homelessness, it was not possible to re-interview potential clients and collect additional information since the screening team was not offering treatment. Often the screening psychiatrist had a one-time only chance to talk with the individual and decide if she/he met the eligibility criteria.

The screening process also encountered the issue of advocacy. A person who was deemed eligible for the study had the opportunity for services, including housing, and if randomized to the ACT team, mobile treatment. Many providers had clients for whom they sought better services. Sometimes there were differences between the researchers and the referring agency regarding interpretation of symptoms and circumstances. Some months into the project it was established that if there was disagreement, the principal investigator retained the final decision to accept or reject a referral. This practice, once established, worked very well. All referrals were given serious consideration. However, it was clearly understood by the provider community that the research team had the authority to make the final decision regarding acceptance into the study.

One problem we had expected was that persons referred to the project would be very guarded and not forthcoming with personal information. For the most part this was not the case. Most individuals were willing to talk with the research team giving detailed accounts of life events and current problems. Rather, the problem for the research team was that if we were unable to accept the individual for the project, how could we make this a constructive process rather than simply another rejection? Most of the people referred were clearly very troubled and were often at a very low point in their lives. Many, particularly those encountered at the night shelters, were not receiving any clinical services at all. While the screening team could not offer any clinical intervention (except when a person was expressing suicidal or homicidal ideation), once it was determined that the person was ineligible for our project, referral to other services were made.

Attrition: Another concern of the research team at the outset of the project was that the attrition rate would be very high. As these individuals were without a stable address or phone number, we anticipated it would be very hard to track them. A strategy we developed to deal with this potential problem was that throughout the project, the same research assistant was responsible for completing all interviews with a subject. This arrangement built trust as well as knowledge of the person's habits and locations. Furthermore, although it was not in the original research design, monthly checklist interviews were added to enable the research assistants to track each individual each month. These interviews took about ten minutes to complete and covered where the person stayed the previous month, service utilization and where we might expect to find them again in one month. The overall follow-up rate for all interviews, except the family interview, remained above 83 percent (many of the participants in the project had lost contact with their family a long time ago and were unable to name a family member who was willing to be interviewed). The combination of the same interviewer at each time point and the frequency of contact facilitated this low attrition rate along with persistence, ingenuity, and good relationships within the homeless provider community.

Informed consent: In this population, obtaining informed consent presented special problems. Many of the participants were actively psychotic and often displayed disorganized thinking at the time of screening. Moving from eligibility to participation in the project took from one to many encounters sometimes spread over a year or more. At the time of consent we had to make sure that all participants understood that:

1) they were signing up for a research study;

2) they had a fifty percent chance of being assigned to the new treatment team;

3) there were housing options available to them irrespective of the outcome of randomization, and;

4) they would have four sets of interviews spread over the forthcoming year for which they would receive $20 per interview.

We learned that to help the individual understand informed consent it was necessary to keep the explanation simple and concrete. In particular, the use of diagrams was often helpful.

Reliability of data: Most of the assessment instruments relied on self-report. This provided certain limitations. While some homeless individuals lead ordered lives, others' lifestyles are very changeable. For many, remembering events in sequence or over long periods was difficult. To enhance reliability, we chose time intervals that were short, no longer than 2 months, and used the monthly checklists to capture residential and service utilization data. In addition, to augment the self-report service utilization data, we used information supplied by the ACT team, Medicaid claims data and data from the client information system maintained by the local mental health authority.

LESSONS LEARNED

Service Intervention

1) Homeless persons with severe mental illnesses are willing to engage in services when they are offered flexibly and persistently.

2) Services must be prepared to address the broad range of client needs including housing, general medical care, legal assistance, financial management, substance abuse treatment, as well as mental health care.

3) Persons recovering from mental illness and/or homelessness can become highly effective members of the service team, acting as a bridge and advocate between the client and the entire service team.

4) Efforts to reach out to families of homeless persons with severe mental illness can be difficult, but when feasible, often bear fruit.

5) Effective advocacy and treatment at times requires the integration of social control mechanisms (for example, representative payeeships, probation) combined with clinical and social support.

Research Component

1) It is possible to conduct longitudinal studies with low attrition rates on very hard-to-track groups such as homeless persons with severe mental illness, provided sufficient personnel, close data management, flexibility, and persistence are applied.

2) In order to recruit a large enough sample, considerable investment of expertise and time is needed.

3) Homeless persons with mental illnesses and the homeless provider community are willing to participate in research as long as the researchers understand and respect their approach/work and all are very clear about the research objectives.

4) If the research design involves testing an intervention, the researchers must be clear that they are not part of the intervention despite their own desires to help and pressure from the service community and subjects to offer assistance.

5) When a researcher is asking a subject to sign an informed consent, the researcher should keep the explanation of the research design simple and ensure that the subject understands all essential parts by asking him or her to repeat or diagram key sections.

REFERENCES

Burns, B.J. & Santos, A.B. (1995). Assertive Community Treatment: An update of randomized trials. *Psychiatric Services* 46:669–675.

Dixon, L., Krauss, N. & Lehman, A. (1994). Consumers as providers: The promise and challenge. *Community Mental Health Journal* 30:615–625.

Essock, S.M. & Kontos, N. (1995). Implementing Assertive Community Treatment Teams. *Psychiatric Services* 46:679–683.

Olfson, M. (1990). Assertive Community Treatment: An Evaluation of the Experimental Evidence. *Hospital and Community Psychiatry* 41:634–641.

Osher, F.C. & Kofoed, L.L. (1989). Treatment of Patients with both Psychiatric and Psychoactive Substance Use Disorders. *Hospital and Community Psychiatry* 40:1025–1030.

Stein, L.I. & Test, M.A. (1975). Alternative to the Hospital: A Controlled Study. I. Conceptual Model, Treatment Program, and Clinical Evaluation. *American Journal of Psychiatry* 132:517–522.

Stein, L.I. & Test, M.A. (1980). Alternative to Mental Hospital Treatment. *Archives of General Psychiatry* 37:392–397.

Teague, G.B., Drake, R.E. & Ackerson, T.H. (1995). Evaluating use of continuous treatment teams for persons with mental illness and substance abuse. *Psychiatric Services* 46:689–695.

Test, M.A. (1979). Continuity of Care in Community Treatment. *New Directions for Mental Health Services* 2:15–22.

Weisbrod, B.A., Test, M.A. & Stein, L.I. (1980). Alternative to Mental Hospital Treatment. II. Economic Cost Benefit Analysis. *Archives of General Psychiatry* 37:400–405.

NOTE

Preparation of this chapter was supported by grant no. 5HD5SSM48070 from the Center for Mental Health Services.

5

Critical Time Intervention for Homeless Mentally Ill Individuals in Transition from Shelter to Community Living

ELIE VALENCIA, EZRA SUSSER, JULIO
TORRES, ALAN FELIX AND SARAH CONOVER

The transition from institutional living to community is a vulnerable and crucial period which challenges the provision of a continuum of care. For homeless people, continuity of care at the time of transition from shelter to community living often results in recurrent homelessness, so that specialized interventions are required.

Critical Time Intervention (CTI) was designed to prevent homelessness among individuals suffering from severe mental illnesses by stabilizing them in the period of transition to living in the community. It seeks to bridge the gap between services for the homeless and community services. The model is specifically designed to complement rather than to parallel the existing service system for mentally ill people in the community.

CTI was tested in a randomized clinical trial between 1990–1994. The site of this clinical trial was the Columbia-Presbyterian Mental Health Program for Homeless Individuals at the Fort Washington shelter for men in New York City (NYC). Preliminary analysis of results indicates that the intervention is effective in reducing recurrent homelessness among mentally ill individuals. CTI continues to be provided at the Columbia-Presbyterian Mental Health Program as an ongoing clinical intervention, funded by the Department of Mental Health of the City of New York.

THE SETTING

The New York City Municipal Shelter System for Men

The scope and severity of homelessness in the City of New York far exceeds that of any other major city anywhere in the United States (Dinkins, 1987; Cuomo 1992). New York City has been under court order to provide shelter to its homeless population for over a decade. (*Callahan v. Carey*, 1981; *Eldridge v. Koch*, 1983; *Thrower v Perales*, 1986). It shelters at least 25,000 individuals during the winter periods. In the last five years, the municipal system has sheltered 5,100 to 8,000 men at any given time (NYC Human Resources Administration, 1989–1992, NYC Department of Homeless Services, 1993–1994).

The demographics of the municipal shelters' male residents has not changed much in the last decade. Most of them are under 40 years old. Men in the shelter system belong overwhelmingly to ethnic minorities, (90%), with a disproportionate presence of African-American (about 70%). Latinos constitute approximately 20%, while Caucasians and individuals of other ethnic backgrounds account for less than 10%. Approximately half of them report that they have been born in New York and have finished high school (Struening, 1988, Cuomo 1992, NYC Department of Homeless Services, 1993–1994). The Fort Washington shelter population is similar to the shelter population at large.

The need for the provision of specialized services for mentally ill individuals in the NYC shelter system has been well documented (Susser *et al.*, 1989; Cuomo, 1992). By 1989, we established that the prevalence of mental illness, excluding substance use, among male shelter dwellers ranged between 20% and 30% (Susser *et al.*, 1989). Among first-time users of the system, on diagnostic interview, 25% had a definite, probable or possible history of psychosis. A recent study indicates that the situation has basically remained the same (Cuomo, 1992). Mental health programs currently operating in the system can at most provide services to about one-fifth of these men. Moreover, these programs are facing budget cuts under the current city and state conservative administrations.

Furthermore, in order to place men in housing for mentally ill individuals, decrease recurrent use of the shelter system and other institutional facilities such as hospitals and prisons, and maintain them in community living, a specialized system of support for the transition period is crucial. Presently, such a system does not exist.

The Fort Washington Armory Men's Shelter

The Fort Washington Armory, located across the street from the Columbia-Presbyterian Medical Center, has been the site of a major municipal shelter since 1981. It is situated in a Latino working class section of Washington Heights in Manhattan. Its population has fluctuated between 200 and 1,000 homeless men in this period. The

Columbia-Presbyterian Mental Health Program For The Homeless has been in operation in this shelter for almost a decade.

At the time of the recruitment of participants for the CTI study, mentally ill persons were haphazardly mingled with hard core substance users and the general population in the Fort Washington Shelter. These men faced a hostile environment. Fort Washington Shelter living placed the most vulnerable residents at a disadvantage. They were often preyed upon by higher functioning residents and/or some custodial staff. Their living conditions were also characterized by neglect, many of them were unable to take care of themselves, and often their personal hygiene deteriorated to the point of infestation. They also had to deal with a high incidence of HIV and tuberculosis infection, as well as with other medical problems (Susser et al., 1993; Susser et al., 1994a; Susser et al., 1994b; Saez et al., in press; Valencia et al., 1996; Valencia et al., 1994).

THE CHALLENGES

Shelterization

In our clinical work over the past decade, we have observed that during the course of a stay in the shelter, men tend to adapt their behavior to conform to institutional living. They are forced to develop the social skills necessary for survival in the shelters. Inadequate staffing, in terms of both numbers and skills, creates a highly volatile environment where violence and abuse of residents is common (Gounis and Susser, 1990, Grunberg and Eagle, 1990). Informal relationships of exchange between staff and residents form a system of privileges and favors which includes some sub-groups and excludes, or even exploits, others (Gounis and Susser, 1990). This system places some of the neediest residents at a disadvantage. These men face a hostile environment where being "successful" in surviving means becoming integrated into the shelter system.

The social skills necessary for shelter living are quite different from those required to survive in the community. For instance, in the shelter there is no need to plan for meals or pay rent, and little privacy is possible. Men become dependent on and accustomed to the limited institutional services provided by the shelter to meet their basic needs. Moreover, with the presence of so many other men within the same four walls, a ready social network is available at any given moment. In the community, on the other hand, in order to live in a Single Room Occupancy hotel (S.R.O.) one must be able to arrange for availability of meals, do laundry, pay rent, form social networks and develop recreational activities. Social isolation may become a substantial barrier to reintegration into the community.

Norms for social behavior in and outside the shelter are in conflict as well. In the shelter it is critical to preserve one's own space. Drug dealing, substance use, "hustling" activities and/or participation in the underground economy are part of the culture and social ecology of these municipal shelters (Susser and Gounis, 1990,

Grunberg and Eagle, 1990). In the community, any of these activities
are likely to get a person thrown out of an apartment, S.R.O. or community residence very quickly.

Thus the behaviors and skills developed for shelter survival make
the transition from shelter into community living particularly difficult for many men, especially for the mentally ill (Susser *et al.*, 1990,
Valencia *et al.*, 1994). To make the transition, a man may be required
to give up his shelter social networks and an environment with which
he has become familiar for an uncertain future in the community. For
some residents, services which address basic daily needs are more
available and integrated in the shelter than in the community, where
service procurement requires planning and coordination. Many men
with long shelter stays have developed high levels of shelterization,
active adaptation to shelter living and inaction, to seek community
based alternatives (Gounis and Susser, 1990). In practice, many men's
stay in the community was short-lived due to some of these factors.
That was the case for many of the men at the Fort Washington Men's
Shelter at the time of recruitment of men for the CTI study.

RECURRENT HOMELESSNESS

By the mid-eighties, in response to the high numbers of people with
mental illness being identified as shelter dwellers, the City of New
York began to fund the development of mental health programs in
the shelters. These programs were designed to meet some of the
psychiatric needs of shelter users while minimizing barriers to use
by providing services on-site. The Columbia-Presbyterian Mental
Health Program was funded as one such program. These programs
provided services to men only during their stay in the shelter.
Services were, and largely still are, discontinued at the time of
discharge from shelter to housing. This constitutes a crucial gap in
the continuum of care of these men. Our experience providing direct
services indicates that men in transition from the shelter have great
difficulties becoming stabilized in the community. We contend that
the need for support services is at a peak at the time of placement in
community housing. However, at this especially vulnerable time,
shelter programs' support services are discontinued while community agencies often are not ready to follow up with the care these
men need.

For these reasons many men return to the shelters or go to the
streets creating a veritable revolving door of homeless recidivism.
An earlier study following up 39 men who were placed in the community by our program strongly indicated the need for supportive
services at the time of transition from shelter based mental health
programs to the community. By 18 months after discharge from the
shelter into community housing arrangements, 41% were again
homeless (Caton *et al.*, 1990, Caton *et al.*, 1993).

We argue that an essential ingredient in a program that could
successfully assist these men in making the transition from the shelter to community is to provide for continuity of services (Valencia

et al., 1994; Susser *et al.*, 1990; Susser, 1990). The evidence accumulated in the area indicates the value and necessity of adaptive long term interventions for mentally ill adults in transition from institutions such as hospitals and shelters to the community (Stein and Test, 1980; Lamb, 1984; Susser *et al.*, 1990). It has also been recognized that the most effective system of care for the chronically mentally ill is through the provision of continuous and lifelong, assertive comprehensive services in the community (Stein and Test, 1985, Witheridge and Dincin, 1985, Harris and Bergman, 1987; Olfson, 1990). However, to the date of this effort the provision of time limited interventions to integrate a continuum of care with existing community services has not been tested.

Based on our clinical experience and our research work, we contend that it is clear that support services at the time of transition to living in the community provide a crucial intervention to meet the specialized needs of mentally ill individuals. Indeed, the time to decrease support is when a person has achieved stability and not when he has just moved out of institutional living. Within this context we developed Critical Time Intervention to address the needs outlined above. Its overriding goal is to help the men create a network based on available community support, both socially and in terms of organized services, which would assist them to re-enter and maintain housing in the community.

IMPLEMENTATION: GUIDING THE TRANSITION

The CTI intervention is designed to bridge the gap between homeless and community services, while complementing rather than parallelling the existing service system for the mentally ill. (Valencia *et al.*, 1994, Susser *et al.*, 1992; Valencia *et al.*, 1996). CTI services are time-limited interventions with a straightforward and highly focused approach that could be replicated with ease (Valencia *et al.*, 1994, Susser *et al.*, 1992; Valencia *et al.*, 1996). The overall goal is to assist each individual in establishing durable systems of support which would outlast the implementation of CTI. Services are provided by a small clinical team (4–6) composed of non-professionals case managers supervised by mental health professionals and with the support of a part-time psychiatrist.

Services are provided in four stages over a period of up to nine months depending on the individual's adaptation and the consolidation of linkages to community systems of care (see Table 5.1). During the course of the intervention the individual moves toward greater autonomy, as community providers gradually assume total responsibility for on-going care.

The Four Stages

CTI services are time constrained and limited to the transition period following discharge to community living. Its implementation

Table 5.1. The Four Stages of Implementation

1. SUPPORT AND ASSESSMENT	a. Development of a treatment plan for the transition b. Intensive support to the patient c. Community assessment visits d. Interim treatment provision by discharging program (e.g. Shelter Mental Health Program) e. Accompanying patient to community referrals
2. NEGOTIATION	a. Identifying potential crises b. Facilitating problem solving/accommodation c. Providing support to patient and providers d. Re-negotiating treatment plan if needed
3. MONITORING	a. Maintaining regular contacts with patient and providers b. Observing how transition plan works c. Intervening selectively
4. TRANSFER OF CARE	a. Reaching a consensus for ongoing support b. Allowing for 1 to 2 months safety net

spans a period of up to nine months post discharge. CTI is carried out in four phases (see Table 5.1) which are:

Stage 1. Support and assessment: In general the CTI team develops a skeleton of the treatment plan before the patient moves into the community. This encompasses the identification of both long-term and short-term issues. Special attention is given to the individual's past history (circumstances which have precipitated housing loss in the past) as well as his current needs. As the period to implement CTI is limited, it becomes important for the team to distinguish between issues which could be addressed immediately, and those which would be passed on to the community supports. The linkages identified are crucial to the success of the intervention. These people or agencies are to assume, gradually, the primary role(s) of supporting the individual in the community.

In the initial phase the CTI clinical team works with patients and community providers to detail treatment plans with specific attention to the five areas of functioning identified as crucial for community stability: medication management, money management, substance use management, crisis management and family support management (see below for details). The CTI team makes detailed arrangements in one or two of these areas which are assessed most critical for the stabilization of the particularly patient (e.g., medication compliance). The emphasis is on establishing support systems that would address the needs of the individual and prove durable – ultimately outliving the nine-month intervention period.

In the first few weeks following placement in community housing, the team maintains a high level of contact with the patient, including visits and regular telephone conversations. The CTI specialist conducts assessment visits to the patient's new residence to evaluate his adaptation to community living. During this phase, interim psychiatric treatment (e.g. medications) continues to be provided through the discharging mental health program (the shelter mental health program) while the CTI specialist identifies people/agencies who would assume coordination of psychiatric aftercare services, including the provision and monitoring of medication. Other relevant aspects of functioning such as money management can continue to be monitored by the CTI team during the transitional period.

Most severely mentally ill patients do not feel comfortable attending a new facility and exhibit little tact in interacting with new and unknown service providers. The CTI team addresses this issue by assisting individuals in developing skills that may enable them to overcome these barriers. For instance, accompanying patients to their respective appointments with new agencies and/or providers serves to alleviate some of this difficulty, while facilitating the development of a linkage.

In this stage the CTI specialist and the patient role-play or practice "in vivo" their tasks relating to their agreed service plan. Initially the CTI specialist functions as the sole liaison between the different supports and the patient. This role is temporary in nature, with supportive services gradually being transferred to community based resources (i.e. community mental health centers, outpatient psychiatric clinics, family, friends, etc.).

Furthermore the CTI specialist assists the new providers in the support network in resolving difficult or conflictive issues. There is potential for tensions to arise as new providers and the patient attempt to adjust to one another. Thus, it is important that a relationship be established between the CTI worker/team and the patient prior to community placement. This foundation enables the CTI specialist to act as a broker – mediating between the individual and his respective networks of support. For example, a compromise worked out in the early phase of adjustment to community living may prevent an eviction or a premature termination of services from a community mental health clinic. This stage of CTI generally spans the initial two months post-discharge. It could, however, be modified depending upon the patient's needs.

Stage 2. Negotiation: The second stage of CTI is devoted to testing and adjusting the systems of support for community living developed in the prior stage. Establishing networks of community support requires negotiation and problem-solving. As the individual adjusts to community living new issues generally arise which necessitate the revision of treatment plans.

In the first month or so of operation of a support system, the CTI team is proactive, identifying potential crises, facilitating problem-solving, and re-negotiating systems as necessary. Identifying problem areas in the patient's transition to the community usually encompasses a range of issues, including medication compliance, substance use, and difficulties which inevitably arise between community providers and patients. Particular attention is directed to those issues which may lead to a housing crisis.

The specialist seeks to facilitate the problem-solving process between the patient and his respective linkages and supports using a variety of approaches. This usually takes the form of a case conference or less formal meetings. In this stage, the specialist continues to act as the primary resource for both parties. Nevertheless, there is less emphasis on direct service during this phase. Fundamental services such as the provision of psychiatric medications, and money management are now provided by community agencies.

For some patients, this period involves a re-negotiation of the treatment plans. In this period new issues often surface which were not addressed in the original treatment plan. Under such circumstances, the CTI specialist, along with relevant providers in the community, would revise the treatment plan. Depending upon the situation, the specialist may be required to initiate new referrals and where appropriate the CTI specialist may involve the patient's new community supports in this process. Subsequently he/she may have to engage in tasks of direct service (e.g., accompanying patients to appointments, assessment visits to a new residence). Any direct service engagement in this phase is to be limited. This stage generally spans over a two month period.

Stage 3. Monitoring: At this point in the intervention, the treatment plan for the transition has been implemented and support systems have been established for the patient in the community. The focus of this stage is to assess whether the treatment goals are proceeding as planned. The emphasis is no longer on direct service, the CTI specialist's role becomes less intensive. The identified providers in the community have assumed primary responsibilities for support services.

The CTI specialist continues to be available for intervention should a crisis emerge or at the request of a caretaker. Regular contact is maintained with both the patient and the providers, but is less intensive than during previous stages of the intervention. Community visits are gradually phased out, with an added emphasis on telephone contact. The team encourages the patient and caretakers to handle emerging problems on their own. In most cases the support system which were established would still need some adjustment in order to be viable in the long run.

This stage of the intervention spans a three month period. This considerable time frame allows for the possibility of a renegotiation of treatment plans should the need arise.

Stage 4. Transfer of care: The transfer of care phase spans the remaining two month period. Preliminary work leading up to the termination is done throughout the intervention. From the onset of the intervention, the CTI specialist assists the patient in securing community linkages which may provide longer-term support. The objective is to stabilize the patient in community living as soon as possible and initiate the transfer of care.

The CTI specialist carries out a series of meetings over a period of two months prior to the projected date of termination. They take place approximately every two weeks. During the course of these sessions, he/she talks to the patient about his feelings concerning termination and attempts to determine precisely how he feels about the different linkages in the relevant areas of intervention.

If the patient is experiencing a particular difficulty in one or more of the areas, the CTI specialist attempts to remedy it by meeting with the person(s) concerned to work out a plan which was to take effect after his/her withdrawal. Finally, he/she meets with the patient and the primary linkage person(s) to "fine-tune" the relationship. A similar plan is implemented for the handling of crises and regular support. The CTI team remains available for consultation throughout this period.

The Five Intervention Areas

The CTI model of services is highly focused. It begins when the patient is ready for discharge into community living and housing placement has been determined. At this time the CTI team gathers data to determine the services needed in one or two of five main areas which have been identified in our clinical work as critical for housing stability in the community (Table 5.2).

Medication management: CTI seeks to provide a focused intervention which emphasizes medication compliance. The CTI specialist aims to establish a system under which a patient can obtain and be encouraged to take his medications. Medication planning requires that as an initial step some basic education is done with the patient: recognition of the dynamics of mental illness and the benefits of medication therapy serve to enhance compliance. Furthermore, an understanding of individual signs of decompensation and/or side effects from medication becomes helpful in offsetting potential crisis situations. A focused intervention with respect to medication involves establishing a feasible plan of accessing and monitoring psychiatric medication. This may involve the participation of a psychiatrist, a pharmacist, a case manager and/or a friend and a relative. All of them play a role in an individualized system to encourage medication adherence.

Money management: In the provision of CTI, money management has been identified as a significant part of the patient's adaptation to community living. The focus is on ensuring that the patient's rent is paid. The CTI specialist "trains" the patient in basic budgeting skills,

Table 5.2. The Five Intervention Areas

1. MEDICATION MANAGEMENT	Focuses on preventing symptom relapse and facilitation of medication compliance.
2. MONEY MANAGEMENT	Focuses on ensuring timely payment of rent.
3. SUBSTANCE USE MANAGEMENT	Focuses on preventing addiction from undermining housing stability, and on encouraging appropriate dual diagnosis treatment.
4. CRISIS MANAGEMENT	Focuses on developing a crisis management plan involving the patient, service providers and informal supports to prevent housing loss.
5. FAMILY RELATION MANAGEMENT	Focuses on providing to families to maintain a modest involvement in the community support network of the patient.

which are then practiced by him in the community. In situations where the individual is unable to master these skills, alternative arrangements are implemented, such as using payees where appropriate.

Attention is also directed towards substance use patterns in relation to money management. For individuals who are struggling to deal with substance use issues, it becomes critical to set up a realistic plan regarding the payment of rent. In the first stage of the implementation of CTI (*Support and Assessment*) monitoring of money management is done by the CTI team. This is transferred to community linkages by the second stage (*Negotiation*). The network of the individuals or resources which can offer support in this area may include a local bank, a landlord, a family member, a guardian, a community residence or other community agency.

Substance use management: Treatment plans with respect to substance use require both long and short term planning. Realistically, during the limited time of the implementation of CTI, the team can only initiate a provisional plan of action in this area. The nature of addiction is such that most individuals require long term support to avoid future relapses. In CTI, the emphasis is placed on identifying agencies and providers which can address these issues beyond the nine-month period. Where appropriate, the CTI specialist aims at motivating patients to enroll in long-term substance abuse treatment programs and providing them with support and linkages for accomplishing this goal. Patients are encouraged to attend outpatient dual-diagnosis/substance abuse programs as needed. All patients willing to attend an intensive substance abuse detoxification program are given appropriate referrals. Furthermore, patients are educated about appropriate informal support networks such as Alcoholics Anonymous or Narcotics Anonymous and encouraged to attend meetings in the community. In addition to such referrals the CTI specialist works with informal supports in the community (e.g., family), educating them about the dynamics of substance use and establishing strategies for their involvement in helping to stabilize the patient.

With substance abusers there is an added emphasis on budgeting and the individual's responsibilities around rent, as outlined in the discussion on money management. Ensuring payment of rent is given precedence in financial planning. Individuals who are coping with substance use issues are at greater risk of losing their housing due to the financial mismanagement which often accompanies addiction.

Housing related crisis management: Crisis situations related to housing involve a range of scenarios, such as a threat of eviction or a psychiatric decompensation. A fundamental housing-related skill is the ability to call on someone to help cope with a crisis. In the implementation of CTI services, the prevention of housing loss requires that the CTI specialist develop a viable crisis plan with the patient which can be implemented beyond the nine-month intervention period. Therefore, the specialist focuses on identifying appropriate community resources for the patient to assist in the prevention of housing loss. In the implementation of CTI, we have found that family supports can play a significant role in this crisis management.

Family support management: CTI encourages patients to maintain relationships with their families when available. The CTI team offers to families some basic psychoeducation about the nature of mental illness and its treatment and trains them in ways to respond to crisis situations that might arise after their relative has been placed in community living. A plan is outlined to facilitate a modest involvement of relatives in the patient's support network, if desirable.

Education for families is provided in meetings at their home when possible. In addition to providing information and support to the parents and relatives of the patient, the CTI specialist seeks to alleviate possible guilt and stigma. As implemented in this population, CTI emphasizes that families are not expected to become the main source of support for the patient but rather it seeks to encourage a modest but crucial role in the overall network of support, such as maintaining regular visits with the patient.

CLINICAL EXAMPLES

In this section, we seek to detail the implementation of CTI services further by drawing on examples from our clinical practice. We utilize some case vignettes to illustrate how the clinical work is carried out in the five intervention stages. For didactic reasons we emphasize one area at a time, although, in our experience two or more may need to be addressed simultaneously. We illustrate how a particular area is dealt with during each of the four stages of the implementation of CTI.

Cases Illustrating Stages on Medication Management

Case 1: "Frank", a 32 year old African American, diagnosed with schizophrenia, was generally compliant with his medication schedule. However, due to his severe substance use problems, he would on several occasions lose his oral medication or plainly forget to take it as prescribed. During the *Support and Assessment* stage the CTI specialist discussed these problems with the patient and his psychiatrist.

The patient was given information about monthly injections. He was persuaded that by receiving his medication via monthly injections he would become more stable with regards to his psychotic episodes. The CTI worker pointed out to the patient that this switch to intramuscular medication would enhance his chances for maintaining permanent housing.

During the *Negotiation* stage, a regular day was scheduled every month for receiving his intra-muscular medication. The CTI specialist informed the staff at his residence and at the dual diagnosis program he attended of this treatment plan. During the *Monitoring* stage the community providers agreed to monitor his compliance and to remind him of his appointments for injections. Sometimes, the CTI specialist would accompany the patient to receive his shot. The patient was encouraged to perform practice runs on his own to receive his injection.

During the *Transfer of Care* stage, in addition to the various formal mental health resources listed above, the CTI specialist enlisted the assistance of key family members; in particular his father was approached as a potential social support. Since it was apparent that the patient's father had a limited understanding of his son's mental illness, the CTI specialist provided him basic psychoeducation about schizophrenia. Afterwards, he was linked to a group for families of mentally ill people to complete his psychoeducational process as well as to receive support in dealing with his son's problem. Throughout this intervention the father played a limited but important role in his son's network of support. This role consisted in visiting and/or contacting him – around the time when he was due for his medication – and reminding him about his injections and positively reinforcing his compliance. Thereafter, the father continued to play that role.

Case 2: Ricardo, a Latino suffering from schizophrenia, had recently learned that he was HIV positive. At first he would discuss the matter only with his CTI specialist and his medical doctor. During the *Support and Assessment* stage he was persuaded to seek out a support group. His CTI specialist obtained a list of groups and spoke to various group facilitators. A group was chosen which matched his particular needs: reflecting his cultural group and persons close in age to him, as well as convenient to his residence.

During the *Negotiation* stage, the CTI specialist explained to the facilitator that because the patient was schizophrenic and had recently moved from the shelter, he might have strong emotional reactions to being in the group and, at times, might demonstrate inappropriate behavior. The facilitator was willing to take this risk and agreed to notify the CTI team of any problem rather than drop the patient from the group.

During the *Monitoring* stage, Ricardo did not want the CTI specialist to accompany him to the group any longer. Thus, he complied with his request. However two weeks later he left the group enraged and insulted and decided not to return. The facilitator immediately notified the CTI worker who in turn notified his psychiatrist and psychiatric nurse, the problem was resolved through case conference and the patient joined the group again three weeks later. He was welcomed back by people who understood his particular situation. During the *Transfer of Care* stage closer psychiatric follow-up was arranged as a backup. The CTI worker introduced the facilitator to the psychiatric nurse by phone and they continued to communicate directly.

Case Illustrating Stages on Money Management

Pedro, a 32 yr. old Latino man, originally from the Dominican Republic with a diagnosis of paranoid schizophrenia, had no benefits when he first entered the program. He was in need of documentation to show he was eligible to apply for benefits. He misused any money which was available to him for the purpose of purchasing drugs and/or alcohol. When he managed to obtain food stamps, he sold them for this purpose. In addition, he used to borrow money from loan sharks at the rate of 200% per week and was seriously threatened when he was late in paying back.

The first step in the *"Support and Assessment"* stage was to help Pedro obtain proper documentation and begin receiving formal assistance. He was sent to re-apply for food stamps, Medicaid, and SSI. When he was approved for this assistance, the CTI team began the implementation of a money management strategy. A savings account was opened for him and his SSI check was deposited.

During the *Negotiation* stage, given the patient's past history of financial mismanagement, an agreement was worked out by the CTI team with Pedro that his mother would be in charge of managing his money. While initially he was somewhat resistant, he acknowledged that this plan would enable him to pay his rent promptly. Also, this plan allowed Pedro to visit his mother on a regular basis and have free meals at her home. A series of sessions were held between members of the CTI team and Pedro's mother to train her in managing his money.

In the *Monitoring* stage, periodic visits were made to their home to monitor money management and provide support for his mother. Finally during the "Transfer of Care" stage his mother was named as payee for his SSI benefits for long-term money management.

Cases Illustrating Stages on Substance Use Management

Case 1: Calvin, a 30 year old Latino man diagnosed with paranoid schizophrenia, was a polysubstance user (heroin, crack, cocaine, marijuana). As a result of intra-venous drug use he became infected with HIV. This led to serious deterioration of his physical and mental health and caused him to contract tuberculosis.

During the *Support and Assessment* stage he attended a Latino support group where he was confronted with his substance use problem. The CTI team recognized a valuable support in his closest friend in the program. The CTI specialist worked with him to persuade the patient to seek help for his substance use problem. He was referred and began attending an outpatient substance use support group in a nearby hospital. Family members were enlisted as community-based supports. This required some education about the dynamics of substance use and strategies for dealing with related behavioral problems or crisis situations. His mother demonstrated a willingness to be involved and agreed to help in monitoring Calvin's substance use.

Home visits were made during the *Monitoring* stage by the CTI specialist and the patient was counselled regularly for his substance use problem, with the goal of persuading him to enroll in a long-term dual-diagnosis program. Ultimately during the *Transfer of Care* he became convinced as to the need for substance use treatment and was referred to an appropriate facility.

Case 2: Hector initially moved to an independent living situation upon leaving the shelter. During the *Support and Assessment* stage it became clear that he needed additional support and was subsequently placed in a supportive SRO. He had a history of heavy crack cocaine use, and relapsed shortly after moving into the SRO. During the *Negotiation* stage the CTI specialist arranged for an assessment and referral to a rehabilitation program. Assistance was sought during the *Monitoring* stage, in determining the appropriate program for Hector through an established community program dealing with substance abuse. Two referrals were made: to a five-day detox facility; and to a longer-term outpatient dual diagnosis program. The referral choice of the outpatient program was carefully selected, as the patient requested a non-confrontational program.

However, this program had a waiting period of one month before Hector could be admitted. Subsequently the CTI specialist worked on identifying community supports for Hector during the interim period. Ultimately during the *Transfer of Care* his worker at his residence offered support to Hector in his efforts to remain drug-free. He entered the outpatient dual diagnosis program following the one month waiting period.

Case Illustrating Stages in Family Support Management

Guillermo, a young Puerto Rican client suffering from schizophrenia, was rejected by numerous community residences because of his substance use problem. He was finally placed with his mother who had expressed her willingness to take him. During the *Support and Assessment* stage the CTI specialist worked through his closest friend in the program to persuade him to seek help for his substance use problem. During the *Negotiation* stage he was referred and began sporadically attending an outpatient dual diagnosis program. In this stage, the CTI team educated his mother about the nature of his son's illness and taught her how to deal with his addictive behavior. The team enlisted her assistance to help in monitoring Guillermo's substance use. The psycho-educational sessions took place at her place and the CTI team made itself available to answer her questions throughout the duration of the intervention.

Two months after placement, Guillermo showed up at the shelter with all his belongings. He stated he had been "evicted" by his mother. He told us she was drunk and simply threw him out. We contacted his mother immediately. It turned out that the client had stolen a few items from the household and showed up early in the morning with a "friend" in a state of acute intoxication, presumably from crack and alcohol use. His mother asked him to leave. She was very upset. His behavior violated the agreement under which the client had been placed, namely to abstain from coming home intoxicated and not to steal from her. Both parties were resistant to talk. Within 24 hours the CTI worker again contacted the mother, and was able to bring the two parties back to the negotiating table. Fortunately, it was Mother's day – a very important day for Latino people – and this contributed to softening their attitude and agreeing to a dialogue. Guillermo apologized and promised to abstain from the behaviors which led to his eviction. He was received back home on the very same day.

Throughout the *Monitoring* stage we visited Guillermo and his mother. We counselled him regularly for his substance use problem with the objective of persuading him to consider enrolling in a long-term dual-diagnosis program. Ultimately, the *Transfer of Care* was achieved and he was referred to the local hospital's program for people with mental illness and chemical addiction which helped him manage his substance use and continued to pursue the goal of getting him to accept long term treatment. The mother also was provided with ongoing support to be able to continue to house his son. Indeed, Guillermo's only alternative to homelessness was to live with his mother – unless he could enter an inpatient long term program for dual diagnosed individuals.

THE STUDY: TESTING THE EFFECTIVENESS OF CTI

The Columbia-Presbyterian Mental Health Program for the Homeless

The Columbia-Presbyterian Mental Health Program for the Homeless served as the basis and the backup clinical program for the implementation and testing of CTI. The program started in 1986 as one of the few mental health programs in shelters which were funded by the City of New York in response to concerns about the prevalence of mental illness among shelter dwellers.

This program provides comprehensive mental health services to mentally ill shelter users, with the goal of engaging them in psychiatric treatment as well as helping them move out to alternative living arrangements in the community (Valencia et al., 1994; Kass et al., 1992; Caton et al., 1990; Valencia et al., 1996). Each year the program provides over 12,000 visits, screens over 400 men and enrolls 150 of them. Around seventy-five men participate in the program at any given time. In a recent survey of 107 program participants, 64 were African-American, 24 Latino, and 8 White and 4 another ethnicity. Thirteen percent were under age 30 years, 45% were age 30–39 years, and 42% were 40 years or older. Seventy percent were diagnosed as suffering from psychotic disorders, mainly schizophrenia. Most of these men are referred to the program by staff of the municipal shelter system, while others are recruited directly by our outreach activities in the shelter.

The program's clinical services are characterized by a coordinated set of interventions grouped into five main clusters of services.

Outreach and engagement: These services are ongoing coordinated social and recreational activities. They are geared to engage the men in the program while carrying out an informal assessment of the strengths and deficits of the individual. They include assertive outreach activities in the shelter for those hard to engage. A core feature of these services is the provision of a supportive and a friendly milieu in the program.

Psychiatric treatment and stabilization: These services include psychiatric evaluation, medication, psychosocial counselling, health maintenance and case management titrated to the needs of the individual. Each individual is assigned a member of the clinical staff as his case manager.

Group activities/Community skills development: These services center around the implementation of specialized groups. They include daily community meetings which provides staff with the opportunity to observe the men for clinical changes. In these meetings, which most attend, the men are encouraged to develop sensitivity to their peers and to the community outside the shelter. Smaller daily living skills groups focus on areas such as hygiene, medication, money management, substance use management and housing alternatives. Also, men are encouraged to participate in recreational and vocational skills development activities and training workshops.

Procurement of entitlements: The program assists all participants to gain access to entitlements, including public assistance, Medicare, Medicaid, and Veterans benefits. Almost all of the men in our program are eligible for, and obtain, SSI benefits.

Housing activities: The program places great emphasis on assisting participants to gain access to existing housing for homeless mentally ill people. Most of this housing is sponsored by the 1990 Agreement of the City of New York and New York State to develop over 5,000 residential units to house mentally ill individuals who are homeless. Our program coordinates and prepares the complete package application to access housing under this agreement. (This application process is time consuming, bureaucratic and burdensome). (Valencia *et al.*, 1994).

Currently almost all the men who complete their on-site treatment plan are placed in community housing within six to twelve months of their enrollment (many within six months or less). The program places about 60 individuals into community living each year. The men move into a wide range of supportive housing, single room occupancy hotels (SROs) with on-site services as well as SROs without services, community residences and adult homes. In addition, some leave to join their families and a few are able to live in shared or independent apartments.

RESEARCH DESIGN

The research design to test the effectiveness of CTI services was a randomized clinical trial. It was tested at the Columbia-Presbyterian Mental Health Program at the Fort Washington shelter for men. Participants were recruited between 1991–1993 among mentally ill individuals being discharged into community living by this program. A total of 102 men were eligible to participate. Ninety six of them consented to participate in the clinical trial. In order to avoid selection bias, participants were randomly selected into experimental and control groups only after housing placement had been selected. Participants in the control group received the usual discharge treatment services offered to individuals enrolled in the mental health program. These services included a comprehensive referral package for continued mental health services in the community, including on-site assistance for three months by the shelter program, when requested. Participants in the experimental group received the CTI services for a period of up to nine months.

Data were collected monthly for 18 months, including comprehensive assessments at baseline, 6 and 18 months. The 18 month follow-up period of the study allowed for measuring concurrent and post-effects of CTI. Since the active period of clinical intervention is limited to nine months, the period from 10–18 months allowed measurement of the lasting effects of CTI. Monthly interviews collected data on homelessness, service utilization and substance use. The comprehensive assessments included evaluation to assess psychopathology, symptomatology, substance use and social functioning. All assessments were blind to the group status of the participants.

PRELIMINARY RESULTS

All 96 participants suffered from severe mental illnesses. They were diagnosed using the Structured Clinical Interview for DSM-III-R (SCID). Most of them have a life time diagnosis of schizophrenia

(69%). Lifetime cocaine abuse were diagnosed in 48%. The majority also suffered from co-occurring substance use disorder. The sample was overwhelmingly composed of men of minority descent (86%): African American men accounted for 69% and Latinos for 27% of the participants. Most of them were in their thirties and had histories of homelessness raging from several months to several years. Recurrent psychiatric hospitalizations and episodes of homelessness were common.

Overall, the characteristics of the two groups at their baseline assessments were similar. However, it should be noted that they differed in three important areas. Participants in the experimental group were more likely to have a co-occurring lifetime diagnosis of cocaine abuse, and were twice as likely to have had more than five or more episodes of homelessness. Men in the control group were twice as likely to have had only on episode of homelessness. Also, the experimental group ended up with six out of the seven study participants who were HIV symptomatic or had AIDS.

The data collection of this clinical trial has been successfully completed. The follow-up rate for the study was very high (98%). Only two of the 96 participants were lost to follow-up, both from the control group. Analysis of the data is still ongoing. However, preliminary results indicate that the intervention is effective. CTI reduced by more than half the average number of homeless nights over the entire 18 months of the study. Also, this preliminary analysis indicates that the effect of CTI remained after it was withdrawn – at least for the remaining 9 months of data collection.

CONCLUDING REMARKS

In this chapter, we have presented a specialized intervention designed to enhance the continuity of care for mentally ill individuals at high risk for homelessness who are discharged from homeless shelters to community living. Existing systems of mental health care for mentally ill people in large urban centers are often fragmented and do not provide for a continuum of care. Difficulties at the point of transition to community living are pervasive in the mental health system in the states.

The transition from shelter living to living in the community is a critical time to establish continuity of care. The provision and development of systems of support in this period are crucial to improve community living tenure. CTI services address these particular needs of mentally ill individuals at risk for homelessness. Preliminary data analysis indicates that it is effective in reducing recurrent homelessness among individuals with severe mental illness. If final results confirm its effectiveness, we believe CTI could be implemented in many programs for mentally ill individuals who are homeless. Moreover, its implementation could be particularly useful for mentally ill individuals at risk for homelessness in transition from other institutional living settings (such as hospitals and prisons) to living in the community.

REFERENCES

Callahan v. Carey. (1981). Index No 4258/79 (Sup. Ct. N.Y. Co. August 26).

Caton, C.L.M., Wyatt, R.J., Grunberg, J. & Felix, A. (1990). An Evaluation of a Mental Health Program for Homeless Men. *American Journal of Psychiatry* 147:3, 286–289.

Caton, C.L.M., Wyatt, R.J., Felix, A., Grunberg, J. & Dominguez, B. (1993). Follow-up of Chronically Homeless Mentally Ill Men. *American Journal of Psychiatry* 150:11, 1639–1642.

Cuomo, A. (Chair) (1992). *The Way Home: A Direction in Social Policy.* Report of New York City Commission on the Homeless, New York City.

Dinkins, D. (1987). *A Shelter Is Not A Home.* Manhattan Borough President Special Report.

Eldridge v. Koch, 98 A.D. 2d 675 (1st Dept, 1983), *rev'g on other grds*, 118 Misc. 2d 163 (Sup. Ct. N.Y. Co. 1983).

Gounis, K. & Susser, E. (1990). Shelterization and its implications for mental health services. In: Cohen N (ed), *Psychiatry Takes To The Streets.* Guilford Press: 231–257.

Grunberg, J. & Eagle, P. (1990). Shelterization: How the Homeless Adapt to Shelter Living. *Hospital and Community Psychiatry* 41:521–525.

Harris, M. & Bergman, H.C. (1987). Case Management with the Chronically Mentally Ill: A Clinical Perspective. *American Journal of Orthopsychiatry* 57(2):296–299.

Kass, F.I., Kahn, D. & Felix, A. (1992). Day Treatment in a Shelter: A Setting for Assessment and Treatment. In Lamb HR, Bachrach LL, Kass FI (eds.) *Treating the Homeless Mentally Ill. A report of Task Force on the Homeless Mentally Ill.* Washington D.C.: American Psychiatric Press: 263–277.

Lamb, R.H. (Eds) (1984). *The Homeless Mentally Ill: A Task Force Report of the American Psychiatric Association.* Washington, DC: American Psychiatric Association.

Olfson, M. (1990). Assertive Community Treatment: An Evaluation of the Experimental Evidence. *Hospital and Community Psychiatry* 41(6):634–641.

New York City Human Resources Administration. (1989–1992). *Monthly Shelter Report.* New York City: Family and Adult Service Division.

New York City, Department of Homeless Services. (1993–1994). *Monthly Shelter Reports.* New York City.

Saez, h., Valencia, E,. Conover, S., Susser, E. (in press) Tuberculosis and HIV among mentally ill men in a New York City Shelter. *American Journal of Public Health.*

Stein, L.M. & Test, M.A. (1980). Alternative to Mental Hospital Treatment, I: Conceptual model, treatment program, and clinical evaluation. *Archives of General Psychiatry* 37:392–397.

Stein, L.M. & Test, MA. (1985). The Evolution of Training in Community Living Model. *New Directions for Mental Health Services* 26:7–16.

Struening, E.L. (1988). *Characteristics of New York City Shelter Residents.* Presented at the First Annual New York State Office of Mental Health Research Conference; December 8: Albany, NY.

Susser, E., Struening, E. & Conover, S. (1989). Psychiatric Problems in Homeless Men: Lifetime Psychosis, Substance Abuse, and Current Distress in New Arrivals at New York City Shelters. *Archives of General Psychiatry* 46:845–850.

Susser, E. (1990). Working with People Who Are Homeless and Mentally Ill: The Role of a Psychiatrist. In: Jahiel R (ed.). *Homelessness: A Preventive Approach.* John Hopkins Press.

Susser, E., White, A. & Goldfinger, S. (1990). Some Clinical Approaches to the Homeless Mentally Ill. *Community Mental Health Journal* 26:459–476.

Susser, E., Valencia, E, & Goldfinger, S.M. (1992). Clinical Care of the Homeless Mentally Ill: Strategies and Adaptations. In Lamb HR, Bachrach L, Kass F (eds.), *Treating the Homeless Mentally Ill* Washington, D.C.: American Psychiatric Association Press: 127–140.

Susser, E., Valencia, E. & Conover, S. (1993). Prevalence of HIV Infection Among Psychiatric Patients in a New York City Men's Shelter. *American Journal of Public Health* 83:568–570.

Susser, E., Valencia, E., Miller, M., Meyer-Bahlburgh, H., Tsi, W. & Conover, S. (1994a). Sexual Behaviors of Homeless Mentally Ill Men at Risk for HIV. *American Journal of Psychiatry* 152(4):583–587.

Susser, E., Valencia, E. & Torres, J. (1994b). A Curriculum for HIV Prevention Among Homeless Mentally Ill Men. *Psychosocial Rehabilitation Journal* 17:31–40.

Thrower v. Perales. (1986). Sup. Ct. N.Y. Co. May 22. Index No 41385/85.

Valencia, E., Susser, E., Felix, A., Caton, C. & Colson, P. (1994). The New York Critical Time Intervention Study: Guiding the Transition to Independent Living, in *Making a Difference. Interim Status Report of the McKinney Demonstration Program for Homeless Mentally Ill.* Adult Center for Mental Health Services Administration. U.S. Dept. of Health and Human Services. April.

Valencia, E., Susser, E. & Goldfinger, S. (1996). Critical Timepoints in the Clinical Care of Homeless Individuals. In Vaccaro J. and Clarke G. (eds.) *Community Psychiatry: Mentally Ill Practioner's Manual.* American Psychiatric Association.

Valencia, E., Torres, J., Susser, E. (1996). Working with Homeless Mentally Ill Men. In Cournos, F. and Bakalar, N. (eds.), *HIV/AIDS and Severe Mental Illness.* Yale University Press.

Witheridge, T.F. & Dincin, J. (1985). The Bridge: An Assertive Outreach Program in an Urban Setting. In: LI Stein, MA Test. (eds.) The Training in Community Living Model: A Decade of Experiences. *New Directions For Mental Health Services.* San Francisco: Jossey-Bass, 26:65–76.

NOTE

Research supported by NIMH/CMHS grant #5R18SM4841-4.We thank the staff of the Critical Time Intervention Mental Health Program for Homeless Individuals, Columbia-Presbyterian Medical Center, at the Fort Washington Shelter for Men in New York City for their contribution to this article. We also acknowledge the contribution of Carol Caton, Ph.D. and Paul Colson, Ph.D. We thank Bibiana Marquez for her administrative support.

6

Supported Independent Housing: Implementation Issues and Solutions in the San Diego Project

RICHARD L. HOUGH, STEVE HARMON, HENRY
TARKE, SANDRA YAMASHIRO, ROBERT
QUINLIVAN, PAULA LANDAU-COX, MICHAEL S.
HURLBURT, PATRICIA A. WOOD, RON MILONE,
VIRGINIA RENKER, ARETA CROWELL and
ELIZABETH MORRIS

The San Diego project was designed to evaluate the effectiveness of providing comprehensive support services coordinated with independent housing (subsidized through Section 8 Certificates) as a method of stabilizing homeless individuals with serious mental disorders in the community. The project was unusual in the level of public/academic collaboration: implementation involved close cooperation among San Diego County Mental Health Services (SDCMHS), San Diego State University, San Ysidro Downtown Mental Health Center, Episcopal Community Services, the San Diego Housing Commission and the Housing Authority of San Diego County. The project was designed to be collaborative in an attempt to address the wide ranging needs of the homeless mentally ill population through interventions that were designed to be responsive to their special needs.

This chapter provides a brief description of the San Diego project and then, in more detail, the kinds of implementation issues that were encountered. Issues arose primarily from two sources: the diverse agendas of the collaborating agencies and the conflicts associated with conducting research in an operating service environment. Contrary to what might be expected, few of the implementation problems stemmed directly from the fact that homeless mentally ill persons (HMI) were the target population for the demonstration project.

RESEARCH DESIGN

The project design was developed to test two current ideas about how people who are homeless and mentally ill can most effectively be served. The first suggests that, with appropriate support, homeless mentally ill people improve their lives significantly when they are provided with access to normal, independent housing in the community (Blanch, Carling & Ridgway, 1988; Carling, 1990; Ridgway & Zipple, 1990; Boydell & Everett, 1992; Carling, 1993; Neubauer, 1993). The second strategy was based on the research literature suggesting that the severely mentally ill can be more effectively maintained in the community with comprehensive case management than with more traditional forms of case management (Stein & Test, 1985; Harris & Bergman, 1987; Bond et al., 1988; Witheridge, 1990).

The general hypothesis was that access to independent housing (through Section 8 Certificates) and access to supportive services in the form of comprehensive case management (CCM), particularly when combined, would produce better client outcomes than lack of direct access to independent housing and more traditional levels of case management. The San Diego demonstration project was designed to test these approaches using a randomized experimental design (Fig. 6.1) where some homeless mentally ill individuals received access to independent housing, some received access to comprehensive case management and some received access to both. Outcomes to be examined included: a) severity of psychopathology; b) stability of housing; c) functional status; d) quality of life and life satisfaction; e) physical health condition; and f) use of mental health services.

Over the first year, the San Diego project received referrals from community programs of some 466 individuals who were homeless and mentally ill. These referrals were screened to identify 362 individuals who were presumed eligible for the study. Final eligibility was determined during the baseline interview at which time clients were randomly assigned to one of the study conditions. The baseline characteristics of the 362 clients have been reported elsewhere (CMHS, 1994), and are briefly summarized here. Approximately two-thirds were male, most were white and most were between 19 and 44 years of age. Total income averaged about $350 per month. Only 10 percent of the clients reported no income, and only 13 percent reported any earned income. The other 77 percent reported entitlement income of some sort. The modal years of education was 12. Approximately one third had been homeless less than one year, one third for between one and three years, and one third for four years or more. The great majority had been homeless more than once and over half had been homeless five times or more. Some

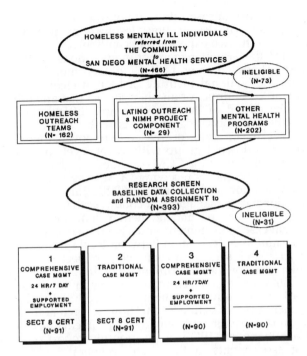

Figure 6.1. San Diego Homeless Demonstration Research Project: Client and Referral Flow

55 percent received a diagnosis of schizophrenia and 45 percent major depression or bipolar disorder. Only 12 percent reported current substance abuse, but approximately 50 percent reported diagnosable abuse at some point in their lives. All but 13 percent had been admitted to a hospital or treatment facility for mental health problems at some point in their lives.

A simple longitudinal factorial experiment was conducted to test the effectiveness of the housing and case management components of the supported housing intervention. Eligible subjects were assigned to one of four conditions formed by crossing the housing and case management variables:

1) CCM with a Section 8 housing certificate;

2) traditional case management with a Section 8 housing certificate;

3) CCM with no housing certificate, and

4) traditional case management with no housing certificate.

Structured interviews took place with all clients at baseline and every six months thereafter for three years, measuring the outcome variables noted above. In addition to the six month follow-up interviews, monthly case manager reports were made for the first twenty-four months and entries in case progress notes were abstracted over the same time period. The design allows testing of the additive and interactive effects of the two experimental conditions.

Originally, the case management interventions in all four conditions were scheduled to end after eighteen months. However, a grant from the National Institute of Mental Health allowed case management to continue for another year so that an additional factor could be added to the study design. Little is known about whether any gains accruing to clients with CCM are maintained when the level of support is decreased or removed; therefore, a transition (or "step down") group with lower levels of case management was established in the CCM conditions. Eighteen months after entering the study, clients receiving CCM were randomly assigned to (a) a continuation of the original CCM for another 12 months or (b) a transitional case management condition that closely resembled traditional homeless case management. Clients originally assigned to traditional case management underwent no change.

The substantial collaboration between local service agencies and university research staff in the San Diego project extended beyond the development of the experimental conditions to the process of collecting information concerning outcomes in the lives of subjects taking part in the study. Staff members at both PHA's kept records of when clients in the Section 8 conditions entered and left Section 8 housing units, reasons for leaving and problems in case management. Case managers filled out a monthly report on each client including assessments of the client's general functioning (e.g., housing, nutrition, grooming, money management), and mental health status (e.g., depression, hostility, self neglect, bizarre behavior, etc.). Agency staff were also continually helpful in locating respondents for follow-up interviews at six month intervals for three years.

FINDINGS

Outcomes from the San Diego Project to date have been described more completely elsewhere (CMHS, 1994; Hough *et al.*, in press; Hurlburt *et al.*, in press) and only a brief overview is reported here. When the housing status of the 362 clients in the San Diego Project were examined at eighteen months into the project, some 60 percent were in independent housing (mostly Section 8 housing for clients in the Section 8 conditions and mostly other independent housing for the non-Section 8 clients), some 20 percent were in community housing (living with friends, family, in group living quarters, etc.), some 10 percent were in institutional housing (hospitals, recovery homes, crisis centers or jails) and less than one percent were in shelters or on the streets. Housing status was unknown for approximately 15 percent of the sample. We estimated that approximately half of the missing were probably homeless. At eighteen months, 148 (82 percent) of the 181 Section 8 condition clients had entered independent housing, and approximately 60 percent of clients in the

Section 8 condition continued to live in independent housing at the end of the 18 months. It appears that CCM was only marginally better than TCM in getting clients into independent housing.

Other Outcomes

Overall, clients in the San Diego Project improved significantly in terms of increases in average monthly income, quality of life scale scores (particularly finances, residence, safety and leisure activities and less so with social relations and physical health), and general health status. Decreases were noted in depression symptom scale scores, the average number of inpatient days, and the percentage of clients with more than two inpatient days in the past 60 days. Generally, no significant differences were found between the case management conditions.

Although most subjects improved significantly on most outcomes examined in the project, few significant differences were found in outcomes between the experimental conditions. Subjects assigned to the Section 8 housing conditions were significantly more likely to express satisfaction with the dimensions of their lives most closely related to housing. In terms of case management effects, however, no significant differences were found between subjects assigned to traditional and comprehensive levels of case management. Interpretation of the lack of differences between case management conditions should not be taken, however, as a general indicator that more intensive levels of case management are not more efficacious with the homeless mentally ill than more traditional levels. It may be, for example, that even more intensive case management with a case goal of 6-10 might be more effective than the comprehensive condition in this project in which there was a case load of 20. Also, it should be noted that the traditional case management program, in this study, was not a general program, but one designed to deal specifically with the homeless mentally ill. The "traditional" program had been in existence for some years prior to the beginning of the research and had a well-trained, seasoned staff with considerable pride in their ability to serve the target population. Further, there was no staff turnover in this program during the project. Conceptually, the lack of differences in outcome by case management conditions could have been due to the exceptional quality of our comparison "traditional" program.

PROBLEMS OF IMPLEMENTATION

The primary focus of this chapter is on the various challenges encountered during implementation of the research design. As suggested earlier, many arose as the collaborating agencies worked to develop an integrated package of services. For example, in the early stages of the study, the formulation of eligibility criteria required compromise among agencies having different operating missions and regulations.

During the delivery of the experimental interventions, competition between case management providers created some problems in maintaining the integrity of the research conditions.

Other implementation problems emerged from the special demands of conducting research with homeless mentally ill people. For example, given the mobile nature of the target population, retaining clients in the research process required constant attention to maintaining the information and social networks that might help interviewers relocate clients.

Negotiation of Eligibility Criteria and Screening Procedures

In general terms, the target population for the project was defined as those individuals who have a primary mental disorder and are homeless or at very high risk of becoming homeless. While these criteria sound relatively straightforward, their operational definitions emerged only after a prolonged negotiation process among the agencies and organizations having a stake in the project. Included among the parties whose interests had to be balanced were the researchers, the SDCMHS administrators, case managers and outreach workers, public housing authority (PHA) administrators, housing specialists and other line staff, and other homeless service providers (e.g., psychiatric hospitals, crisis centers, mental health centers, transitional housing programs, and shelters).

The need to balance the interests of various stake-holders resulted in a narrowing of eligibility criteria. Several of the participating service agencies operate under local, state, and/or national regulations that define their scope of responsibility and the clientele they are to serve. SDCMHS, the provider of the case management programs, does not serve persons with primary diagnoses of substance abuse or those on probation. By state policy, clients with primary substance abuse problems are to be served by county alcohol and drug treatment programs and individuals on probation must have their public mental health services provided by the state probation system. The two PHAs that administered Section 8 certificates have different regulations designed to protect the rental housing in which their clients are placed and to protect the neighbors of clients. For example, clients cannot be dangerous to themselves or others and must have a source of income to contribute to the rental costs. Each of these restrictions excluded some clients from participation, but all three agencies worked closely together to modify and stretch their service eligibility criteria to accommodate the special characteristics of this population. Even in a highly collaborative environment, however, there still were problems with defining eligibility requirements with regard to the definition of primary mental illness and homelessness, and with handling prior alcohol and illegal drug use, and prior criminal behavior.

The eligibility criteria that emerged from negotiations among all interested parties and the research staff are summarized in Table 6.1. Despite the strong pressures to select a narrow sample of individuals generated by different agency guidelines, the flexibility of participat-

Table 6.1. Eligibility Criteria.

---

1. Persistent, primary major mental disorder, in a non-acute phase at time of referral. (Usually operationalized as a current DSM-III-R diagnosis of Schizophrenic, Bipolar or Major Depressive Disorder on the Diagnostic Interview Schedule (DIS). In the absence of a DIS based diagnosis, a few clients with incontrovertible evidence of diagnosis were admitted.)
2. Not a danger to self or others. (e.g., client is not in need of crisis intervention. Client is also past any crisis phase and no serious homicidal threat or suicidal ideation is evident.)
3. Has not been arrested for the manufacture or sale of illegal drugs.
4. If has a recent history of illegal drug use, is actively committed to a drug-free lifestyle and is working toward recovery.
5. Has not been arrested for any *felonious* violent criminal activity that has as one of it elements the use of force.
6. Is homeless – undomiciled and does not reside at a fixed address designed for or ordinarily used as a regular place of residence.
7. If in a public or private shelter or transitional program, has lived consecutively in such accommodations 45 days or less by time of referral.
8. Able to live independently with supports.
9. Eligible or potentially eligible for some income that would allow the individual to maintain an apartment.
10. Owes no money to a public housing authority.
11. Willing to participate in the research and accept case management services for at least 12 months.

---

ing agencies allowed a subset of the population to participate in the study that may well be a representative of those most likely to be eligible for many public services.

Development of Referral and Screening Procedures

Subject recruitment is a special problem for any research project dealing with mental illness and homelessness. The San Diego project recruited subjects through referrals from homeless shelters, other programs that target the homeless mentally ill and local public mental health programs.

Table 6.2 summarizes the number of clients referred from different sources. Some 466 potential subjects were referred by homeless outreach teams, emergency psychiatric units, case management services, outpatient programs, socialization centers, day treatment centers, regional outpatient clinics and crisis residential centers. Just over half of the referrals came from programs within the SDCMHS, with an additional 191 from county contract programs and only 20 from other sources. A special Hispanic Outreach unit provided 33 referrals. Hispanic populations are consistently reported to under-utilize

Table 6.2. Sources of Referrals

SDCMHS		Contract Programs		Other	
Regional homeless outreach teams	180	Crisis centers	80	VA Homeless Outreach	11
Hispanic Outreach	33	Mental health center	80	Transitional housing programs	5
Case and program managers	17	Day care programs	13	Private practice	2
NIMH homeless coordinator	13	Hospitals	9	Hospitals	2
Psychiatric hospital	12	Transitional housing programs	6		
		Medical care and social Service Centers	3		
TOTALS	255		191		20

outpatient mental health services (Hough *et al.*, 1987; Wells *et al.*, 1987; Kulka *et al.*, 1990) and that pattern has been true for SDCMHS over the years. The degree to which under-utilization results from different cultural perspectives concerning mental health, lack of knowledge concerning how to access mental health systems or other barriers to utilization is not clear. To encourage more Latinos to participate in the San Diego Project, a full time Hispanic outreach worker was hired. As a result, Hispanics comprised 12.5 percent of the total sample of clients enrolled in the project, a significant improvement over the 7 percent of the HMI typically observed in SDCMHS services. Hispanic women were, however, particularly difficult to recruit.

Potential clients for the study were screened for eligibility at three stages. First, personnel in the referring organizations informally selected those individuals in their service populations who might meet project eligibility criteria. The 466 individuals passing this first screen were then reviewed by telephone by the research project director to determine whether eligibility criteria were met; 73 individuals were excluded at this stage. The remaining 393 individuals who passed the telephone screen took part in a baseline interview to assess eligibility using standardized protocols.

Special Problems in Implementing the Eligibility Criteria

Identifying the primary mental disorder: It was relatively easy to establish agreement on the general definition of a primary mental disorder such as schizophrenia or a major mood disorder, persistent in duration, and severe enough to cause behavior dysfunction such as substantial interference with primary activities of daily living with need for rehabilitation services for an indefinite period of time. Disagreement emerged as researchers, referral sources and case managers tried to implement the definition, in many cases arising from differences in the agendas of the research team and the referral sources. Referral sources tended to be more liberal than research staff in their definition of major mental disorders. Generally, they were anxious to get their clients into the project in order to provide them with the opportunity to obtain housing and other services, as well as to lighten their own case loads. Unfortunately, this led some referral sources to over-emphasize the severity of mental illness in some cases and to over-estimate the ability of other clients to live in independent housing.

Three procedures were adopted to deal with this problem. First, training sessions were developed for referring programs and agencies to help them understand that the project could only admit subjects who were seriously mentally ill, but not so ill that institutional care was needed. Second, shelters and other homeless service programs that did not have internal means for accurately assessing the mental health status of clients were directed to the regional homeless outreach teams who provided an initial mental health evaluation. These "indirect referrals" appear under the category of "regional homeless outreach team" referrals in Table 2, but account for no more than 15 percent of their referrals. Third, the Diagnostic Interview Schedule (DIS), a standardized instrument described later in this chapter, was used as the final screening tool for the presence of serious mental disorder for all subjects.

Identifying homelessness: Numerous situations arose where staff from the referral agencies, the research team and the public housing authorities disagreed on whether a person met the homelessness criterion. Problems in deciding whether a person was homeless occurred at referral, during research screening and during the PHA Section 8 application process.

At the referral stage, differences of opinion about the definition of homelessness arose between referral sources and research staff members. Referral sources were typically interested in advocating for their clients and tended to adopt a more liberal definition of homelessness than did the research team. This was particularly true given the incentives the project created in the community. Getting clients accepted in the research project allowed the referral sources to feel they had obtained valuable services for their clients, lightened their caseloads, and provided the clients with the possibility of receiving Section 8 certificates – highly valuable in San Diego's expensive housing market. Project entry also ensured rapid access to Section 8 certificates, in comparison to being placed on the standard four year waiting list. For these reasons, referral sources, at times, wished to refer into the project clients who were living in difficult or highly tenuous situations, such as a client living with an emotionally abusive mother or a client who had been a long term resident of a shelter and was about to be released. In response to such problems, the project eligibility criteria were broadened to include referrals if they had lived consecutively in a public or private shelter or transitional program 45 days or less at the time of referral and if they were in imminent danger of becoming homeless upon leaving the program. Disagreements occurring at the point of project referral sometimes created time lags in referral acceptance which, in turn, created problems in working with mobile individuals who were not always easily re-contacted once eligibility decisions were made. This was a continual problem that only resolved itself through experience and time.

Other disagreements concerning implementation of the homelessness criteria arose between the research team and PHA staff. Disagreement focused primarily on how literally the homelessness criteria were to be applied at the time the client was applying for Section 8 housing. The HUD definition of homelessness at the start of this project was:

> "Any individual or family who lacks a fixed, regular, and adequate nighttime residence; and has a primary nighttime residence that is: a) A supervised publicly or privately operated shelter designed to provide temporary living accommodations (including welfare hotels, congregated shelters, and transitional housing for the mentally ill); b) An institution that provides a temporary residence for individuals intended to be institutionalized; or c) A public or private place not designed for, or ordinarily used as, a regular sleeping accommodation for human beings."

PHA Section 8 eligibility review staff initially interpreted this definition very conservatively and were reluctant to accept as homeless any client who was currently or had recently been residing in a shelter, treatment program, jail or other institutional setting. Referral sources and research staff tended to interpret the definition more liberally and to classify as eligible individuals who were at immediate risk of homelessness. These "at immediate risk" subjects included, for example, persons who had reached the limit of housing allowances in a given shelter or treatment program and who had no known financial support or housing available through other programs, family or friends. Additionally, case managers in the San Diego Project often placed individuals temporarily in shelters until the Section 8 process could be negotiated. When PHA staff evaluated these subjects for Section 8 admission they often did not regard clients temporarily residing in shelters as literally homeless.

Two solutions were worked out. First, it was agreed that PHA staff would accept a case manager's written certification that his or her client was "homeless". In reference to "at-immediate risk" clients, the research screening staff and case managers were allowed to define individuals as eligible for the project in cases where the threat of homelessness appeared imminent. Second, homeless status was designated to apply at the point of project entry and not at the point of Section 8 application. By accepting the time of entry into the program as the definitive point for judging eligibility, clients temporarily placed in shelters by project case managers were able to obtain Section 8 certificates.

Illegal drug use: Whether illegal substance abusing individuals should be allowed into the project was another significant issue, with differing perspectives held by the researchers, PHA authorities and case managers. The intent of the original design was that, within reason, clients with some substance abuse problems were to be included. However, federal regulations issued in the month immediately preceding project implementation threatened the achievement of this objective. On the basis of these regulations, one of the local public housing authorities strengthened its zero tolerance policy on illegal drug usage. The primary intent of the new regulations was to exclude from Section 8 eligibility those persons who had been involved in illegal drug usage within one year of intake.

Due to their recent issuance, these regulations had not been fully operationalized when the project began. Numerous issues arose regarding their implementation, for the project clients as well as for the general Section 8 population. For example, the policy excluded individuals who had been *arrested* for illegal drug possession. Many felt the exclusion on the basis of arrest, as opposed to conviction, was a violation of the civil rights of applicants. Of more importance to the research design, strict application of the zero drug tolerance policy would have excluded a large proportion of homeless mentally ill people, among whom the prevalence of substance abuse is very high.

As a compromise, the local PHAs agreed to accept into Section 8 housing, on a case-by-case basis, persons who had recent histories of illegal substance abuse or arrest for abuse, if they were committed to recovery and were involved in a treatment intervention. Judgments about use, commitment to recovery and probable project eligibility were first made by the referral source. Further assessment of substance abuse patterns and commitment to recovery were made in the telephone screen and, finally, substance abuse among potential subjects was assessed in the baseline interview. After the decision to admit, the case manager's judgement concerning the client's level of commitment to recovery and involvement in treatment were accepted by the PHAs as proof that the substance abuse criteria were met. Individuals with a history of arrest for sale or manufacture for sale of illegal substances were screened out of the study.

While the PHA authorities were ultimately satisfied with the procedures described above, case managers consistently felt that individuals with a primary diagnosis of substance abuse were inappropriate for the study and that they were often not successfully identified by the DIS. In a few cases, clients turned out to be serious drug abusers with no willingness to commit to treatment. While the possible admission of individuals whose primary diagnosis was alcohol abuse or dependence was not of great concern to the PHA authorities, this possibility was of great concern to case managers because these individuals were seen as the clientele of San Diego County Alcohol and Substance Abuse Services and not of this project.

Criminal behaviors: HUD regulations excluded from Section 8 housing individuals with a history of arrest or conviction for a felony that involved the use of violence or force. While there was general agreement that a recent felony conviction involving violence or force was a reasonable exclusion criterion, it was debated how serious the violence should be, whether "arrest" alone should be reason for lifetime exclusion from eligibility for Section 8 housing. In this case, the resolution adopted was that unless an applicant was found to have committed a recent seriously violent or forceful crime, criminal records would be reviewed on a case-by-case basis to determine eligibility for admission. In a few cases, for example, clients who had used a weapon in a car theft or some less serious crime twenty or thirty years before and had no criminal record since were admitted. As with substance abuse, the resolution of this problem was that PHA authorities agreed to accept the recommendation of the case manager concerning the client's eligibility. However, following HUD regulations, individuals having an outstanding debt to a public housing authority were also excluded.

The overall "balancing of risk": A very difficult judgement call in the screening process was whether a client was capable of independent living and appropriate for case management. A balance had to be maintained in the project between taking only "good clients" who were very clean in terms of criminal and substance abuse histories and taking clients who were much more risky. One purpose of the research was to test the extent to which a program relying on PHA certificates for independent housing and mental health case management resources could be used to deal with a HMI population, even when substance abuse and/or criminal behavior complicated the picture, while acknowledging that clients who were too prone to violent or illegal behavior could jeopardize case managers and neighbors. Balancing those two concerns necessitated more careful screening than some potential clients and referral sources might have preferred and assigning to case management some clients who case managers might have traditionally preferred to exclude.

As noted earlier, clients were screened for program admission at three stages. The reasons for screening out individuals at each stage are shown in Table 6.3. For example, referral sources said, on average, that they excluded 33 percent of the HMI receiving services in their program because of serious drug abuse with no apparent intent to seek treatment. The other major reasons for exclusion included mental disorders other than schizophrenia, major depression or bipolar disorder, lack of capacity to live independently, and failure to meet the project homelessness criteria. Referral sources estimated that some 9 percent of those they asked if they wanted to enter the project refused the offer.

Random Assignment

The fact that subjects were randomly assigned was problematic to many referral sources and clinical staff. The former simply wanted to

Table 6.3. Reasons for Screening Subjects Out of the Project, by Screening Agent

	Screening Agent		
	Referral Source (percent)	Telephone Screen (number)	Research Interview (number)
1. Serious drug abuse	33	7	2
2. Recent history of selling drugs	5	0	0
3. No appropriate mental disorder	23	17	7
4. Not capable of independent living	22	5	0
5. Do not meet homeless criteria	18	13	3
6. Client Refusal	9	4	0
7. History of arrest for violent crimes	8	20	10
8. On parole	5	3	1
9. Alcohol abuse primary	0	4	2
10. Cannot complete interview*	0	0	5
11. Duplicate	0	0	1

* Subjects who were functionally unable or who were decompensating so badly that they were unable to complete the interview.

obtain the best possible treatment for their clients. Clinical staff were typically more accustomed to having the authority to determine what levels and types of service their clients were to receive. Initially and periodically throughout the project, both referral agents and case managers had difficulty accepting the fact that, as a result of random assignment, some clients were assigned to conditions in which they had access to Section 8 housing even though they didn't really want it or would not make use of it, while other clients who had a strong desire for such housing would be assigned to conditions with no Section 8 access. The solution to this problem was to provide training sessions for the referring agencies in which the project goals and procedures were presented. For clinical staff, similar training and case manager debriefings in which they were encouraged to discuss their feelings about the project were provided. Most clinical and referral source staff accepted the randomization process when they realized that all clients received some increased services, and that the program was viewed positively by most clients, regardless of the mix of services received.

Care was taken to make sure that the vulnerability of the homeless mentally ill person was taken into account in the randomization procedure. First, it was recognized that random assignment had to take place simultaneously with completion of the baseline interview to prevent loss of subjects. Therefore, research interviewers were given a summary sheet that helped them to determine if the client met criteria for a primary psychiatric diagnosis and for homelessness at the close of the interview, at which time a sealed envelope immediately identified the treatment group assignment and provided specific written instructions as to how the client was to proceed. To make sure there was appropriate support and counseling for clients screened out of the project by the baseline interview, all baseline interviews were conducted in locations where a referral source representative could join the client and the interviewer as the results of the interview were shared.

Implementation of the Case Management Conditions

In both the CCM and TCM conditions, the research design called for case managers to provide both direct services to their clients and linkage to other available services to address a wide range of specified needs.

Although both groups of case managers addressed similar types of client needs, the two conditions differed on several dimensions (Table 6.4). Both were administered and monitored by SDCMHS staff, however the CCM component was operated by a private, not for profit, provider under contract with the County. The TCM component was operated directly by the County using staff from their ongoing case management program for the homeless. The contract for the comprehensive program and the County operated program were administered by different individuals within SDCMHS.

As the table shows, the CCM program's staff to client ratio was approximately twice that of the TCM program and CCM case managers were much more accessible than TCM case managers in terms of service hours. Clients in the CCM condition had access to case management services seven days per week, 24 hours per day, as opposed to clients in the TCM condition who had access only Monday through Friday from 8 a.m. to 5 p.m. To further facilitate access to case management services, CCM clients were able to use an "800" telephone number that provided free, direct access to case management services at all times.

Table 6.4. Service Component Comparisons

	CCM	TCM
1. Caseload Size	22 Max	40 Max
2. Team Approach	Yes	No
3. Client Access to Services	7 Days/24 hrs	5 Days/8 hrs
4. Intake	Immediate	7–14 Days
5. Housing Support Groups	Yes	No
6. Specialized Training	Yes	No
7. Service Brokering Funds	Yes	No
8. Supported Employment	Yes	No

Rather than use the traditional individual approach to case management, which involves a relationship between the client and a single case manager, staff members in the CCM condition took a team approach to the delivery of services in which all team members knew each other's clients. Case managers met daily for client updates and brainstorming sessions where ideas were generated on how best to service clients. When a client's regular case manager was not on duty, the team approach made it possible for someone with knowledge about him or her to be available at all times.

CCM case managers also provided some services not available to clients in the TCM condition. For example, intake was immediate, some service brokering funds were available to CCM case managers to purchase needed services and CCM case managers could refer to a supported employment program financed by project funds. CCM case managers also provided, on an "as needed" basis, support groups for clients entering independent housing. CCM case managers received specialized training in the use of an intensive case management approach and on working with the substance abusing mentally ill. Finally, case managers in the CCM program developed start-up kits consisting of basic household supplies for clients moving into their apartments and a food pantry available to clients also on an as-needed basis.

In addition to the services directly provided by the two case management programs, case managers in both the CCM and TCM conditions had access to the entire public mental health service delivery system. All case managers were also able to access substance abuse programs and to work with providers to acquire other services such as food, clothing, furniture, physical health care, and dental services.

Implementing the Case Management Conditions

Most of the implementation problems had to do with the new working conditions the research project introduced into the case management programs. For example, the intervention models called for case managers to work more directly than usual on the substance abuse and employment issues of their clients. Being part of a research project also created some strain for case managers by removing their control over closing cases, by requiring more "paperwork" and by requiring their cooperation with research staff and interviewers. Problems were also encountered in keeping the two case management conditions as distinctly different as they were meant to be. Each of these problem areas is discussed more completely below.

Substance abuse: Clients with substance abuse problems were an especially difficult, ongoing, problem in the San Diego Project. Estimates of the prevalence of dual diagnosis within the homeless population range from 10 to 20 percent (Drake, Osher, & Wallach, 1991) to 50 percent (Tessler & Dennis, 1989). Individuals dually diagnosed with substance abuse and mental illness are often the most difficult to work with. They tend to be less able to manage their lives in the community, show greater hostility, suicidality and speech disorganization; have poorer medication compliance, and are more likely to be re-hospitalized during one-year followup (Drake & Wallach, 1989) (Schmidt, 1992).

In the San Diego Project, approximately 30 percent of clients reported current alcohol or drug use at baseline. Just over 50 percent of the subjects admitted problematic substance abuse at some previous point in their lifetime. Undoubtedly, however, both the current and lifetime admission estimates were low, given the incentives to deny use in order to meet eligibility criteria. Informal case manager feedback suggests that a 50 percent current use rate was probably more accurate for clients admitted to the project.

Clients who were dually diagnosable during the project or who had a history of substance abuse but were currently in recovery presented special problems to case managers, mostly in the areas of community adjustment, independent living, and compliance with mental health treatment and medication. Most case managers had little or no formal training to work with dually diagnosed homeless clients and few had experience of serving them in the community in a case management framework. What is more, they also indicated their greatest resource problem was finding psychiatrists or other mental health professionals who could help manage co-morbid clients.

Several strategies were developed to deal with this problem. In the comprehensive case management component of the program, a dual diagnosis training program was arranged with the help of SAMHSA staff and the National Resource Center for the Homeless. Training was provided by the Dartmouth Psychiatric Research Center in New Hampshire. The training program was conducted in small groups, was based on actual practice situations and focused on how case managers can serve the dually diagnosed living in community settings.

Case managers in the traditional component did not participate in the specialized training described above, since the research design dictated that their program approximate normal service delivery patterns as closely as possible. However, other strategies were developed to effectively serve these clients. One approach was to begin combining case management services with court ordered conservatorship. In California there are provisions in the Welfare and Institutions Code that permit individuals to be placed on a mental health conservatorship if they are found to be unable to provide for their own food, shelter and clothing. In such circumstances, the Superior Court will designate a conservator to oversee the rights and medical treatment of conservatees. In most cases, the Department of Social Services Public Conservators Program is named the conservator.

Case managers in the traditional program began to work cooperatively with staff from the Public Conservatorship program to serve their clients. Via an interagency agreement, case managers provided all mental health services and treatment, while the Public Conservator's staff enforced the legal requirements of the conservatorship. This arrangement allowed case managers to commit clients for involuntary psychiatric treatment when it was clinically indicated. The leverage given the case manager by this power was used to assist clients in maintaining sobriety. Case managers report that having this type of authority has successfully reduced extended hospitalizations. Other recent research (Lamb & Weinberger, 1993) has indicated the clinical effectiveness of this approach.

Another difficulty confronted case managers in their work with dually diagnosed clients. When significant substance abuse problems were detected, the case manager often faced a potential compromise of confidentiality. Maintaining the client's right to confidentiality conflicted with the case manager's responsibility to certify for the PHA authorities that clients in the Section 8 program met eligibility requirements by either not using illegal drugs or by seriously trying to quit and actively pursuing treatment.

Vocational rehabilitation: Initially the CCM team worked closely with a supported employment component (Project Breakthrough) that was contracted to a separate agency. Clients in the CCM conditions who expressed a desire to be involved in vocational services were referred to Breakthrough, which provided trained employment specialists to assist with job readiness, job selection, placement, on site training and coordination with employers. However, the vocational component had major difficulties in attracting and maintaining clients. Some 72 of the 181 CCM clients participated in vocational orientation sessions, 45 formally enrolled in the component and 9 were able to find competitive employment during the initial 19 months of the program.

After careful consideration, it was decided that most of the subjects in CCM appeared to be at a pre-vocational level. Most clients needed to focus their time and effort on taking care of housing, financial and personal issues. Any needed vocational services could be provided directly by the case managers. The Project Breakthrough contract was terminated after a NIMH site review supported the same conclusions.

Competing case management and research concerns: A set of practical problems encountered in this project revolved around the need for the service providers to operate within research constraints and for the research staff to recognize the need for working within the specific service agency's constraints.

The ultimate control for the policies and procedures to be used in service delivery in a demonstration research program have to be driven by research considerations. At times, this became a management issue for program managers with staff who had never before worked in a research-designed service delivery program. On a day-to-day basis, the staff of the service program are surrounded by other case management programs that operate independently and set the expectations and norms within which the research program case managers tend to see their work. In particular, four problem areas were particularly troublesome and involved considerable time and resources to negotiate.

Case load considerations: The research design specified case load size for the CCM and TCM conditions, random assignment of subjects to those conditions and that cases would remain open until the close of the project. Case managers, especially in the TCM condition, were used to having some control over the assessment of their clients, decisions about admission to case management and decisions about the appropriate point in time to close a case. The research project specifications for case management procedures removed their control over these decisions. In this case, the competing demands of case management and research were relatively easily resolved by continuing education concerning the goals of the project. Case managers were also encouraged to give feed-back to research staff concerning the appropriateness of clients being accepted into the project and were given the freedom to minimize their attempts to deliver services to clients who had been placed on parole or who became too threatening or volatile, even though the case remained open.

Additional paperwork problems: Case management staff on this project had additional paperwork requirements as compared to their co-workers in other case management programs. Forms pertaining to the clients' functioning were submitted to the research team on a monthly basis. During the course of the project, County Case Management changed their record keeping and case file documentation practices in a manner that significantly lessened their documentation requirements. Unfortunately, the decreased documentation of the case management process threatened the ability of the research team to continue abstracting case files. Since an important goal of the research was to describe what case managers do, it was decided that case managers in this program would continue documenting their interaction with clients in the original manner. Case management program staff working on this research project were therefore unable to make these changes that would have significantly decreased their workload.

Mental health assessment at program entry: The disagreements between referral sources, case managers and research staff concerning the appropriate mental health status for project entry should be noted briefly here. Case managers in the TCM condition were accustomed to screening their intakes and determining who would enter their program. In order to make sure that standardized, consistent and reliable screening was achieved, the design for the project had research staff conduct standard screening on all potential intakes to determine their entry into the project. This sometimes led to case managers working with clients with whom they would not normally have worked in their previous assignments. Case managers tended to define appropriate criteria more narrowly than the research team, particularly in cases where both major depression and substance abuse were present. As noted above, the solution to this problem was to screen as carefully as possible for cases in which major depression was primary. The problem remained salient, however, throughout the length of the project.

Research interviewer/case manager interaction: Two extremely competent interviewers conducted nearly all the research interviews and are to be credited with the excellent completion rates in the project (nearly 85 percent through the 18 month followups). However, the interviewers' need to maintain positive relationships with the project clients in order to assure high retention rates sometimes led to conflicts over their appropriate roles, particularly in relation to the case managers. The high followup success rate can be attributed to the degree of rapport and level of trust between interviewer and clients. Interviewers were trained not to try to provide services and to concentrate on remaining as objective as possible in their administration of the standardized interview instruments. However, without conveying a sense of caring for the respondents, tracking and interviewing them over three years would have become extremely difficult. At times, interviewers were able to maintain contact and rapport with clients when relationships between the client and case manager had become strained or had even ceased to exist. Under these conditions, interviewers often found themselves in the awkward position of listening to a client's expressions of dissatisfaction with living arrangements, medical treatment or life in general and, sometimes, to a client's appeals for help from the interviewer. Under such conditions interviewers were trained to encourage the client to call their case manager. The interviewers were obligated to inform case managers, with or without client permission, if health or circumstances appeared to put the client or others at serious risk for suicide, homicidal behavior, or life threatening illness.

Given these kinds of interactions with clients and case managers, the interviewers were sometimes viewed as interfering with the normal practice of case management, particularly for the TCM condition in which case managers carried a heavy case load and knew they were supposed to be maintaining "normal" levels of case management. Not only did interviewer provision of information about clients and client provision of information concerning their relationships to the interviewers add to the work load of the case manager, but also sometimes created a feeling of loss of control over "their" client.

Problems in this area were, however, relatively easily contained by maintenance of daily communication between the service program managers and the research office. Interviewer activities were constantly reviewed to maintain the fine line between being researchers and client advocates.

Potential competition between clinical programs: An ongoing problem in the project was the understandable desire of case managers in the TCM component not to "look bad" in comparison to case managers in the CCM condition. After all, the TCM program had been designed precisely to serve the target population of homeless mentally ill for the SDCMHS. Considerable month to month attention had to be given to making sure case managers in this program did not get so competitive that they began to seriously alter the traditional case management program control group function they were slated to perform in the research design. This situation was monitored through monthly meetings with the TCM and CCM program managers and weekly by the TCM coordinator and case managers. Given the constraints of large case loads in the TCM and careful management, no significant changes in TCM work patterns were observed.

In sum, in a service program that is part of a formally evaluated demonstration program, service staff may have difficulty adjusting to the fact that service delivery is not their only responsibility and that they may have less freedom than usual to determine what clients are to receive what services for what period of time. In this project, management had repeatedly to assist staff to accept the fact that the project was research driven and that the delivery of services needed to occur within research guidelines in order to assure that there would be useful and interpretable results.

Implementation of the Housing Conditions

Integration of mental health and housing services: Implementation of the housing component of this project necessitated the "marriage" of three distinct public entities – the local public mental health system and two local public housing authorities (PHAs). Each entity has its own set of extensive and frequently cumbersome regulations, which sometimes made it difficult to refer clients between the systems. The San Diego project was fortunate to work with administrators and staff in each of the three agencies who were deeply committed to making an integrated set of services work to serve the needs of the target population and who were therefore willing to negotiate and to push the limits of their usual operating procedures to make the system work. Negotiation and compromise were particularly needed in reference to Section 8 application and processing procedures, defining "homeless populations," policies concerning illegal substance use and policies concerning criminal behaviors. The latter three areas all required negotiations between the public agencies concerning eligibility criteria for the clients of the intervention.

Section 8 application and processing procedures: In order to maximize access by project participants to the Section 8 program, a "user-friendly" process was negotiated with the two PHAs. Modifications made in the PHAs standard procedures to accommodate some of the special needs of the project's target population included: a) assignment of responsibility for all NIMH project participants to one specific housing specialist; b) streamlining of the Section 8 intake process (e.g., briefing on Section 8 rules and regulations, obtaining all necessary documentation prior to processing); and c) leniency in enforcement of rules related to areas such as missed appointments and length of time available to locate a rental unit.

Location of appropriate housing: Once clients were qualified for Section 8 housing, problems were encountered in selecting appropriate placements. For example, if clients chose to live too close to the same geographic area in which they had been homeless, they ran the risk of being drawn back into the old social networks and behaviors that may have helped to reinforce their homelessness. If, on the other hand, the client was located too far from familiar neighborhoods and from friends, the risk was that isolation and disorientation might complicate the adjustment process. A balance also had to be reached between being close to services, in affordable housing and location in high risk environments. Finally, client preferences in location sometimes had to be balanced with the difficulty of living independently in environments without appropriate supports. Extensive case management involvement in the entire process was required to appropriately balance these considerations.

Dealing with client adjustment to housing: Once clients were in housing, the comprehensive case management component developed housing support groups run by the case managers to deal with the isolation experienced by clients who had lost the support network that the streets had offered. Once in Section 8 independent living apartments, some clients felt very isolated. Their days that used to be consumed with solving the issues of where they were going to get a meal, a hot shower, and a place to sleep that evening, were left with few activities and little direction. For a few of these individuals, returning to the streets was the chosen resolution. The support groups were designed to facilitate clients' transition from homelessness to stable living, to increase their opportunities for successful integration into society and to assist clients in regaining control of their lives by introducing them to a new support system of friends. A specialized support group evolved which focused on the transitional problems of substance abusing clients. The groups, however, did not maintain the participation of clients over more than a few sessions and served relatively few of them.

Retention

Sample maintenance is an important matter in any longitudinal study. It was anticipated that it would be an especially difficult problem with a homeless mentally ill population. However, the San Diego Project was able to maintain an 85-90 percent retention rate over 18 months and 80 percent completions through 30 months. Several factors help to account for this success. First, the availability of case management and/or housing stabilized the lives of a large proportion of clients and, because they have remained in stable housing and in contact with their case managers, they have been relatively easy to track.

Second, the research staff put in place a number of procedures that helped to keep track of clients and to keep them positively disposed toward the project:

- information was gathered in every interview as to where the respondents might be found for subsequent interviews and who might be able to help find them;

- the interviewers initiated a tracking log in which they recorded any information they picked up from other clients, caseworkers, and friends or family of the client about the whereabouts of the client and their future plans;

- a $20 reward was provided for a completed interview;

- with appropriate cautions for interviewer safety, interviewers completed interviews in physical environments comfortable for the respondent (e.g., fast food restaurants, parks, in their cars, public libraries);
- awards (certificates) for participation were provided;
- holiday greetings were sent;
- interviewer business cards were regularly distributed to make sure the project phone numbers were known to clients;
- a toll-free telephone number was provided to allow clients to contact the research office at any time of the day or night;
- an interviewer tracking and appointment system was developed so that any research office staff member could make at least a tentative appointment for an interview with the client;
- interviewers carried beepers to remain in constant communication with the research office in order to respond to requests for interview appointments or changes as quickly as possible;
- county social service and jail records were regularly checked for project client names;
- phone interviews were completed with respondents currently living outside of San Diego County;
- interviewers spent a few days each month combing the streets and other areas frequented by missing clients.

Third, two full time interviewers were with the project from the beginning and became extremely well known to the homeless communities in San Diego County, as well as to service agency personnel who deal with the homeless. Their networks made the tracking of missing clients more feasible than might be assumed. Both were also "street wise," willing to work odd hours and to interview in many difficult situations.

CONCLUSIONS

The San Diego McKinney Homeless Demonstration Research Project was designed to determine whether access to independent housing with case management support services would be an effective method for stabilizing the HMI. This chapter has described many of the problems the San Diego researchers found in implementing the randomized experimental design. Some of the problems encountered were due to the difficulties inherent in recruiting and retaining a homeless mentally ill population in longitudinal research designs. The problems of recruitment were largely resolved in this project by the use of SDCMHS homeless outreach workers and social service agencies as referral points.

Perhaps the greatest difficulties stemmed, however, from the fact that the needs of the HMI cannot be met without providing coordinated, simultaneous access to a wide range of services that are provided by a number of public service agencies, each of which has its own set of guidelines and its own priorities. Problems were often encountered in establishing definitions of the target populations (the "homeless" and the "mentally ill") and in implementing the agreed upon definitions in recruitment, screening and selection procedures.

The most important strategy used to overcome these challenges was the early recruitment of top administrative officials from the concerned organizations into project leadership. Their commitment to making the collaborative project work enabled us to surmount most of the problems faced.

Perhaps the most remarkable aspect of this project has been the level of cooperation between SDCMHS and the PHAs. The initial commitment by leaders of these systems to make the project work enabled the provision of coordinated housing and mental health services resources by project participants. Certainly, the project outcomes suggest that similar cross-agency demonstration and service programs can be launched on behalf of the homeless mentally ill in communities with sufficient will and cooperative spirit to overcome the inevitable bureaucratic and organizational barriers.

REFERENCES

Blanch, A.K., Carling, P.J. & Ridgway, P. (1988). Normal housing with specialized supports. *Rehabilitation Psychology* 33:47–55.

Bond, G.R., Miller, L.D., Krumwied, R.D. *et al.* (1988). Assertive case management in three CMHC's: a controlled study. *Hospital and Community Psychiatry* 39:411–418.

Boydell, K.M. & Everett, B. (1992). What makes a house a home? An evaluation of a supported housing project for individuals with long-term psychiatric backgrounds. *Canadian Journal of Community Mental Health* 100–123.

Carling, P.J. (1990). Supported housing. An evaluation agenda. *Psychosocial Rehabilitation Journal* 13:95–104.

Carling, P.J. (1993). Housing and supports for persons with mental illness: Emerging approaches to research and practice. *Hospital and Community Psychiatry* 44:439–449.

CMHS. (1994). *Making a Difference: Interim Status report of the McKinney Demonstration Program for Homeless Adults with Serious Mental Illness.* Rockville, Maryland: Center for Mental Health Services.

Drake, R.R., Osher, F.C. & Wallach, M.A. (1991). Homelessness and dual diagnosis. *American Psychologist* 46:1149–1158.

Drake, R.R. & Wallach, M.A. (1989). Substance abuse among the chronically mentally ill. *Hospital and Community Psychiatry* 40:1041–1045.

Harris, M. & Bergman, H.C. (1987). Case management with the chronically mentally ill: A clinical perspective. *American Journal of Orthopsychiatry* 57:296–302.

Hough, R.R., Landsverk, J.L., Karno, M., Burnam, M.A., Timbers, D.M., Escobar, J.I. & Regier, D.R. (1987). Utilization of health and mental health services by Los Angeles Mexican Americans and Nonhispanic Whites. *Archives of General Psychiatry* 44:702–709.

Hough, R.R., Tarke, H., Renker, V., Shields, P. & Glatstein, J. (in press). Recruitment and retention of the homeless mentally ill in research. *Journal of Consulting and Clinical Psychology.*

Hurlburt, M.S., Hough, R.L. & Wood, P.A. (in press). The mediating effects of substance use problems on supported housing for the mentally ill homeless. *Psychiatric Services.*

Kulka, R.A., Schlenger, W.E., Fairbank, J.A., Jordan, B.K., Hough, R.R., Marmar, C.R. & Weiss, D.S. (1990). *Trauma and the Vietnam War Generation: Report of findings from the national Vietnam Veterans Readjustment Study.* New York: Brunner/Mazel.

Lamb, H.R. & Weinberger, L.E. (1993). Therapeutic use of conservatorship in the treatment of gravely disabled psychiatric patients. *Hospital and Community Psychiatry* 44:147–150.

Neubauer, R. (1993). Housing preferences of homeless men and women in a shelter population. *Hospital and Community Psychiatry* 44:492–494.

Ridgway, P. & Zipple, A.M. (1990). The paradigm shift in residential services: From the linear continuum to supported housing approaches. *Psychosocial Rehabilitation Journal* 13:11–31.

Schmidt, L. (1992). A profile of problem drinkers in public mental health services. *Hospital and Community Psychiatry* 43:245–250.

Stein, L.I. & Test, M.A. (1985). *The Training in Community Living Model: A Decade of Experience. New Directions for Mental Health Services.* San Francisco: Jossey-Bass.

Tessler, R.C. & Dennis, D.L. (1989). *A synthesis of NIMH-funded research concerning persons who are homeless and mentally ill.* Rockville, MD: National Institute of Mental Health, Division of Education and Service System Liaison.

Wells, K.B., Hough, R.R., Golding, J.M., Burnam, M.A. & Karno, M. (1987). Which Mexican Americans underutilize health services?" *American Journal of Psychiatry* 144:918–922.

Witheridge, T.F. (1990). Assertive community treatment as a supported housing approach. *Psychosocial Rehabilitation Journal* 13:69–75.

NOTE

Research supported by the National Institute of Mental Health and Center for Mental Health Services grants # MH48095.

7

The Effectiveness of Psychiatric Rehabilitation for Persons who are Street Dwelling with Serious Disability Related to Mental Illness

DAVID L. SHERN, SAM TSEMBERIS, JIM WINARSKI, NANCY COPE, MIKAL COHEN and WILLIAM ANTHONY

Individuals with mental illness who are street dwelling present several public policy and service dilemmas. Their rejection of traditional services, coupled with their difficulty in gaining access to many desired resources, makes engaging and serving this group particularly challenging. While increased government funds may be used to improve availability of services, innovative service delivery strategies are also required. For three years, our research group has been involved in implementing and intensively studying an experimental program that was designed to test several propositions regarding how best to deliver services to this group. The rationale for the program reflected our experience, our understanding of the literature, and our analysis of the shortcomings in the existing service system in New York City.

Implementing the research demonstration was extremely difficult owing to both the characteristics of the service population and the New York City environment. In this paper we recount the most important challenges that we faced in developing, implementing, and studying this experimental program. First, we will detail the rationale

for the intervention and its overall design. Then we will discuss its
implementation and the operation of our program model, the Choices
program. We will end by highlighting some of the major findings
from the study from both qualitative and quantitative perspectives.

RATIONALE FOR THE EXPERIMENTAL INTERVENTION

Based on our analysis of the weaknesses of the current treatment
system in New York City and the needs of this federally funded
research demonstration, the experimental program was designed to
meet three criteria: it had to be generalizable, emphasize client
choices, and maximize continuity and accountability.

Generalizability

First, to produce generalizable knowledge, the intervention had to be
replicable and well codified. For over 15 years, members of our
research team have been developing, studying, and disseminating
psychiatric rehabilitation technology (see Anthony, Cohen, and
Farkas 1990). This technology has been demonstrated to affect positively a broad range of outcomes for individuals with mental illness
(Dion and Anthony 1987). We hypothesized that the philosophy and
values that underlie this technology would be responsive to the needs
of homeless people. The approach is well codified: Manuals and training materials are available for all of the major components of this
technology including connecting with consumers, service planning,
linking consumers to service providers, assessing readiness for
rehabilitation, developing readiness for rehabilitation, setting self-
determined rehabilitation goals, performing functional assessments,
and providing direct skills teaching (Cohen, Danley, and Nemec 1985;
Cohen, Farkas, and Cohen 1986, 1992; Cohen, Nemec, Farkas, and
Forbess 1988; Cohen, Farkas, Cohen, and Unger 1990; Cohen and
Forbess 1993). This codification, as well as the well-organized dissemination resources at the Boston University (BU) Center for Psychiatric Rehabilitation, helped to assure that a successful program
could be replicated. Finally, although the technology has been shown
to be effective in a large number of studies, it has been criticized as
only appropriate for individuals who function well and represent traditional middle class values. Testing it on an inner city, largely minority population allowed us to assess its broader applicability.

Choice-Driven Program Philosophy

The second criterion for the program related to its values and philosophy. Individuals who are homeless and who have psychiatric
disabilities are very difficult to engage in traditional services
(N. Cohen, Putnam, and Sullivan 1984). Their rejection of services
may be based in part on experiences with a system that does not

meet their self-defined needs (Barrow 1988). There is evidence that individuals will accept services that are responsive to their self-defined needs (Tessler and Dennis 1989) and that place more emphasis on meeting basic needs than on addressing mental health concerns (Struening 1986; Plapinger 1988). Other authors have discussed specific modifications of clinical and case management programs to more successfully engage and serve this population that often include client definition of needs, long engagement periods, more emphasis on client advocacy, and less role differentiation between helper and client than would traditionally be the case (Freddolino and Moxley 1992; Susser, Goldfinger, and White 1990).

We designed the program to emphasize client choice as the central organizing principle. We reasoned that an idiographically oriented program, stressing client direction and definition of needs, would be more successful at engaging and serving this population than would one emphasizing normative behavior and more prescribed approaches to treatment and support. The program, known as Choices, stressed client direction of the rehabilitation process through both the definition of goals and the selection of appropriate skill and support interventions. The program also included flexible resources and a physical plant designed to meet the immediate basic needs of individuals for food, respite housing, showers, storage lockers, telephones, and laundry facilities.

Structural Continuity and Accountability

The final criterion involved the program's structure. We hypothesized that the segmentation in the New York City service system is an important impediment to successful use of services by street dwelling persons with mental illness. The system in New York includes several components that are loosely organized, often through informal arrangements. For example, an individual who is living on the streets may be first identified and contacted by a street outreach team that may work with the individual for weeks to months to establish a rudimentary relationship. Following successful engagement, the individual may be encouraged to attend a drop-in center or to begin using a public shelter. At the drop-in center, the prospective client may meet a case manager who is associated with the program. The case manager may begin the process of obtaining entitlements and accessing housing and may refer the individual to a clinic, day treatment program, or psychosocial club where the treatment process can begin.

From the client's perspective, therefore, the standard service system in New York City involves a series of transitions between caregivers and programs. These transitions are often not accompanied by a continuity of relationship in caregiver or program. This system segmentation requires individuals who are often profoundly disaffiliated from other persons as well as from the formal treatment system to negotiate access to several systems, each with its own idiosyncratic eligibility and enrollment process.

We reasoned that negotiating each of these transition points in the system without a continuous advocate would be an arduous task for anyone, but especially for individuals who had rejected and been rejected by the traditional treatment system (N. Cohen and Tsemberis 1991). We wished, therefore, to design an experimental program that emphasized continuity in the relationships between the client and his/her caregiver from engagement on the street through ongoing support in getting and keeping permanent housing. Providing this continuity, we hypothesized, would increase the likelihood of long-term engagement and community reintegration.

Another structural feature of the research demonstration program also significantly differs from standard treatment. Standard system designs typically create treatment capacity and identify general target populations without singling out particular individuals for service. Given state reimbursement systems that reward client contacts rather than outcomes, programs are likely to preferentially serve the more engageable individuals in the street population. In contrast, staff of the demonstration program had to establish contact with and follow participants who often were not interested in being followed. From our experience with the Intensive Case Management program (Shern, Surles, and Waizer 1989), we hypothesized that a single point of accountability for each client was an important structural feature of the demonstration program that would complement its structural continuity.

The research demonstration program then was based on a core technology and philosophy of psychiatric rehabilitation that seemed likely to be responsive to the experiences and needs of the street population with mental illness. Given this group's rejection of traditional approaches and their difficultly in traversing the segmented treatment and support system, we hoped that a client-directed program that emphasized continuity in relationships and basic survival and support services would be more successful than the standard treatment system in New York City.

FEATURES OF THE PROGRAM

The experimental intervention was developed and implemented through the Choices program. The program has four major features: outreach and engagement, the Choices Center, respite housing, and follow-along coordination of on-site rehabilitation and support. The design of the program is based upon a core set of three principles. The first is that persons served by the program are capable of making choices and that, to the degree possible, their choices will form the basis of their individual rehabilitation plans. The second is that all individuals need skills and supports to be successful in meeting their goals. The program assures that these skills and supports are provided. It also seeks to develop natural sources of support rather than relying solely on formal services. Finally, for those individuals who are attempting to reintegrate into a social system and who are likely to be suspicious and alienated, the program provides continuity of relationship from outreach and engagement through program graduation.

Although not formally part of the program, Choices was designed to access specialty housing for persons who are homeless and mentally ill that was developed under a special city/state initiative. To address the shortage of affordable and acceptable housing in New York City, the City and State of New York entered into an agreement in 1989 to develop 3,300 new units of specialty housing for individuals who are homeless and mentally ill. The type of housing stock constructed under the agreement has been diverse, with a primary emphasis on permanent housing offering flexible support services. Most of the sites are single-room occupancy (SRO) buildings with 24-hour front-desk coverage and on-site services. Approximately 500 supported housing rental units are included in the State contribution to the total of over 5,000 housing settings. This housing stock was available to participants in both the experimental and control conditions and provided a critical resource required for the success of our experimental program.

Outreach and Engagement

Study participants were identified and screened by research interviewers. For participants assigned to the experimental condition, interviewers coordinated an introduction to rehabilitation staff either on the street or at the program site. Following this introduction, the rehabilitation staff attempted to engage experimental group participants in the program. Standard engagement techniques were used, including the provision of food, cigarettes, and clothing, and assistance with contacting agencies or family members, etc. These engagement strategies were offered as low-demand attempts to begin a conversation with the individual and to establish regular contact. After establishing a rudimentary relationship with the individual, the staff member invited him/her to attend the Choices Center.

On average, individuals in the experimental program received slightly more than five outreach visits. Of the 91 individuals who were randomly assigned to the experimental condition, 80 received outreach services and 75 attended the Choices Center at least once. Choices had a low client-to-staff ratio. Given research attrition, the effective caseload was approximately 13 clients per rehabilitation specialist.

Choices Center

The Choices Center is modeled after successful drop-in centers and provided the primary point of contact with project staff. It was staffed by a team leader, five rehabilitation specialists, a secretary/receptionist, a floor manager, a volunteer coordinator, and a variable number of respite staff who oversaw the respite housing program to be discussed below. Additionally, a part-time public health nurse and psychiatrist visited the program regularly. The Center was open every day from approximately 7 AM through 7 PM.

Only experimental subjects were permitted to use the Center where showers, lockers, laundry facilities, a small library, personal computers, a television and VCR, and telephones were available. As with the outreach component of the program, the Center was low demand and required no program participation. However, for those individuals who chose to participate, three major types of activities were available: (1) assistance with obtaining needed health, mental health, dental, and social services including help with procuring entitlements, (2) development and implementation of an individual rehabilitation plan with special emphasis on housing, and (3) provision of opportunities to meet and develop relationships with other individuals attending the Center.

Respite Housing

For those individuals who chose to leave the streets, housing was provided in small, informal church-based shelters or in blocks of rooms rented by the program at the YMCA. This respite housing was staffed by volunteers from churches and by Choices respite staff who accompanied the clients to the housing and spent the evening with them. Approximately 18 individuals per night participated in the respite housing program throughout the first 16 months of program operation.

Follow-Along, On-Site Rehabilitation and Support

For those individuals who obtained community housing, Choices rehabilitation specialists continued to work with them by providing follow-along and on-site services to continue implementation of their rehabilitation plans. Each plan involved a careful assessment of the services and supports needed by the individual to achieve his/her goals. The rehabilitation specialist assured that these resources were available and provided skills training as indicated. Follow-along, therefore, provided complete continuity of care by staff from the streets through permanent housing.

RESEARCH METHODS

The clinical trials methodology used in conducting this research demonstration involved identifying potential participants in the research on the street through either referral from homeless outreach programs or through direct observation by interviewers. Once provisionally identified as eligible for the study, individuals were screened, informed consent was obtained, and random assignment to either the experimental Choices program or to standard treatment was made. For the experimental group, research interviewers were responsible for introducing the prospective clients to the rehabilitation specialists from Choices. We followed these subjects for 24 months and attempted to collect service utilization and housing data from them every two weeks.

Subject Identification and Recruitment

This task proved more difficult than projected and required a full year to complete. We initially planned to receive all research referrals from Project HELP, the mobile emergency and outreach team operated by the New York City Health and Hospitals Corporation and managed by one of the project co-investigators (Tsemberis, N. Cohen, and Jones 1993). The HELP program, staffed by psychiatrists and other mental health professionals, evaluates and maintains a database on over 3,000 individuals with mental illness who are homeless. Although a large number of individuals were known to the HELP program, its staff was unable to routinely locate and identify them. We were thus forced to expand our recruitment network to include other outreach teams and drop-in centers. Additionally, interviewers began to screen and recruit subjects directly into the study from the streets. Approximately 56% of research participants were directly recruited into the study, with the remaining 44% being identified through referrals. Subjects were continuously entered into the study over the one-year period.

Subject Eligibility and Screening Procedures

Five eligibility criteria were used in the study, operationalized through a structured screening protocol administered by well-trained research interviewers. First, the individual had to have spent at least 7 of the last 14 days on the street. This included sleeping in any space not designed for overnight accommodations. Second, the individual had to evidence psychiatric problems either by self-reporting or being observed to have two mental health symptoms or by having a probable DSM-III-R Axis I or Axis II diagnosis as reported by Project HELP staff. Individuals who were exclusively diagnosed with an alcohol or substance abuse disorder, developmental disability, or organic brain syndrome were not permitted to participate in the study. Third, the individual had to either report disability related to mental illness or be judged by the interviewer or a collateral to evidence a psychiatric disability in hygiene, medical care, nutrition, employment, or social support. While we originally planned to include a criterion related to duration of disability, we were unable to do this because we could not successfully operationalize it in the field. Additionally, the individual had to be judged not to be dangerous to self or others and had to be older than 18.

Four-hundred ten persons were screened and 308 individuals were found to be eligible for the study. Approximately 12% of the screened subjects did not meet symptom or diagnostic criteria while an additional 8% did not meet disability criteria. Only one subject was found ineligible owing to dangerousness.

Subject Consent and Assignment to Condition

Of the 308 individuals who met criteria for inclusion in the study, 174 individuals (56%) completed the informed consent procedure and agreed to participate in the study. Of these, 168 completed the full baseline questionnaire. Participants were generally representative of individuals eligible for the study, with any biases favoring a slightly more symptomatic and male research sample. Ninety-one individuals were assigned to the experimental group and 77 to the control condition. Experimental subjects were introduced to Choices staff by their interviewers while control group members were given information regarding locally available homeless services.

Data Collection Strategy

Subject-specific data were collected in four ways. Two involved highly structured interviews: the Service Utilization Questionnaire and the Baseline and Follow-up interviews. To help us stay in contact, we attempted to interview subjects every two weeks with the Service Utilization Questionnaire. The Baseline and Follow-up interviews were scheduled to occur at six-month intervals, with individuals eligible for reinterview within two months of their six-month anniversary.

In addition to these structured interviews, data were collected from experimental subjects and program staff through unstructured, detailed interviews that were conducted by a qualitative researcher (Lovell and Cohn, in press). Special studies were also undertaken to assess the fidelity of model transfer from BU to the Choices program (see Shern, Trochim, and LaComb 1995) and to assess the characteristics of the standard treatment condition (see Lovell, Richmond, and Shern 1993).

Measurement Model

Four major domains are included in our measurement model. which is depicted in Figure 7.1. Measures of the program intervention were obtained through qualitative research and management information systems at the experimental program. Subject characteristics, mediating variables, and outcome measures were included in the structured research interviews. A more detailed description of the measures included in the study may be found in Shern (1993).

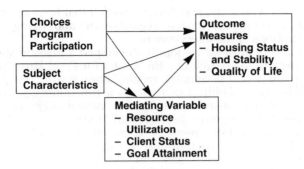

Figure 7.1. Logic and Measurement Model for Hypothesized Client Outcomes.

Baseline Description of the Sample

The research sample is primarily male (76%), black (61%), and non-Hispanic (90%). On average, individuals in the sample are 40 years old (ranging from 21 to 66), unmarried (75% single), unemployed (97%) with over half of the sample (52%) being high school graduates. Over 50% of the sample has been homeless for over four years. Clinically, 75% of participants report that they have had a psychiatric hospitalization. SCID-S diagnoses (Spitzer, Endicott and Gibbons 1992) conducted on a sample of 57 participants indicated that 42% had a diagnosis of schizophrenia, schizoaffective disorder or other psychotic disorder (NOS) while 31% had affective disorders. DSM-III-R Axis V Global Assessment of Functioning scores (mean = 41) indicated serious to major impairment. Over 50% of the subjects met criteria for an alcohol/substance abuse or dependence diagnosis at some point during their lifetime.

DEVELOPING THE PROGRAM

Reaching Consensus on Project Mission and Values

The first challenge confronted by the project leadership was to use the psychiatric rehabilitation technology developed at the Boston University Center (Anthony, Cohen and Farkas, 1990) to define and implement a client centered rehabilitation program. We decided that while not all project leaders needed to be experts in rehabilitation, it was important that all have a working knowledge of the philosophy, principles, and facts on which psychiatric rehabilitation is based. We explicitly created consensus on the program's mission and fundamental principles. This agreement on philosophical issues served as a guide for resolving a variety of implementation questions (e.g., program features, outcome measures, staff selection). In addition, since the project involved such a decentralized management group

(Albany, New York City, and Boston), we felt that it was critical that everyone be "on the same page" regarding the underlying rationale and assumptions of the intervention.

To begin this process, we jointly developed a mission statement for the program. As defined by the Center for Psychiatric Rehabilitation, the mission of psychiatric rehabilitation is to "... help people with psychiatric disabilities increase their functioning so that they are successful and satisfied in their environment of choice with the least amount of ongoing professional intervention" (Anthony, Cohen and Farkas 1990, page 2). These environments have been broadly characterized as living, learning, working, or social. As would be expected, this project's initial focus was the living environment of choice. However, in the McKinney grant proposal, the mission statement's environmental focus had been modified to read "... successful and satisfied in the housing of their choice ..." (Shern 1990, page 60). It was this word changed from living environment to housing environment that became a major source of discussion because of its implications for the program intervention and the research outcomes. If the program was to be consistent with the psychiatric rehabilitation mission, then whatever living environment the participant chose (including continuing to live on the streets) would be an acceptable option to the program staff. They would work with the participants on their terms and honor their choices. However, a major hypothesis of the research was that the experimental group would be more apt to reside in community housing. Yet, if the psychiatric rehabilitation intervention was implemented true to its principles, individuals would have to be fully served even if they did not desire to move to community housing. In other words, people would be helped to become more successful and satisfied no matter what living environment they chose.

The issue was resolved by writing the Choices program mission statement to be consistent with the psychiatric rehabilitation mission. The mission statement was written to focus on "... satisfaction and successful functioning in the living environments of choice." We believed that, once successfully engaged in the program, only a few people with mental illness would prefer to continue to live on the street. Also, if people who chose to remain on the streets were helped by the program, changes on outcome measures other than community housing would occur (e.g., quality of life).

Our discussion highlighted a core issue in the project – that of honoring the individual's choices. While on one level this is an easy principle to endorse, it becomes more difficult when a person's choices seem to be counter either to the major objectives of the project or to ordinary notions of good judgment. Our decision, however, was consistent with the core rationale for the program intervention that emphasized client direction as an engagement and service strategy.

The resolution of our differences regarding the mission statement exemplifies the problem-solving approach that was adopted by our management group. We attempted to use consensus management, which was guided by the values underlying the psychiatric rehabilitation approach. Using this problem-solving technique helped to guarantee that the program was implemented as intended in order to provide a fair test of the effectiveness of psychiatric rehabilitation in this setting.

Staff Selection

We selected Choices staff in a very systematic manner using written protocols to assess the applicants' attitudes, knowledge, experience, and skills. The attitudes identified included valuing client choice and involvement, having an outcome orientation, and having tolerance for diversity and compassion for others. Knowledge and experience in areas such as programs for individuals who are homeless, substance abuse/addiction, psychiatric disabilities, street outreach, crisis intervention, case management, advocacy, the New York City service delivery system, public benefits, housing, and residential programs were assessed as were the applicants' basic literacy, ability to negotiate New York City public transportation system, and research documentation skills. Specific knowledge of psychiatric rehabilitation technologies was also examined.

We believe the screening process was effective for selecting qualified candidates. Over 24 months, we retained four of the original seven rehabilitation specialists. We believe that only one staff person left owing to poor selection procedures or a mismatch between training and the psychiatric rehabilitation approach. In hindsight, we would have weighted experience with alcohol/substance abuse more heavily to assure adequate staff skills in this area.

In addition to the selection of the rehabilitation specialists, we also employed a group of paraprofessional staff to work with program participants, whom we came to refer to as members. Initially, this staff was used to run the respite housing program. They met with program participants in the early evening and accompanied them to the churches where we ran a small 10-bed respite housing program. Respite staff would assist with the preparation of the evening, stay with the members during the evening, and bring them back to the Choices Center in the morning. For these positions we hired individuals who were formerly or currently homeless – many of whom were in recovery from alcohol or substance abuse disorders. As with the criteria for selection of the rehabilitation staff, we also evaluated the candidates for respite positions for their endorsement of the psychiatric rehabilitation values.

Critical Rehabilitation Practitioner Activities

Our analysis of the tasks that the rehabilitation specialists would have to complete led to the identification of the key activities for which they would be responsible. These activities were sequenced and began with the initial engagement of people living on the streets and proceeded through skill and resource development activities

for persons who had obtained permanent housing. The rehabilitation specialists were taught the skills necessary to conduct each
activity competently. Activities during an initial contact included
assessment of survival status, crisis intervention, development/
implementation of a connecting plan, intake into the program, and
provision of basic supports. The specialist's objective was to meet a
participant's most immediate needs for survival and to begin to
develop a trusting relationship that would form the foundation for
future interventions. During this initial phase, the program member
typically began to make use of the Choices Center, including its food
and clothing resources, showers, lockers, and respite housing program. Program members were never required, but always were
encouraged, to participate in all of the activities.

When a program member achieved an adequate level of stability
relative to basic survival and had begun to develop a relationship
with a rehabilitation specialist, an assessment of rehabilitation readiness was conducted. This provided us with information about the
participant's interest in and capacity to participate in a process of
choosing, acquiring, and maintaining a living environment. The
rehabilitation specialist determined whether the program member
needed and wanted to participate in any of the following services:

1. Case management activities focused on linking the member to
   essential services.

2. Psychiatric rehabilitation activities that focused on developing
   the members' skills and supports necessary to attain desired
   goals.

3. Readiness development activities that focused on enhancing each
   member's capacity to become involved in the process of setting
   and realizing a goal.

Rehabilitation Specialist Training

Based in part on our analysis of the key rehabilitation specialist
activities, we structured a three-month training program in which we
emphasized both the skills of psychiatric rehabilitation and those
required to work with this population of individuals who were street
dwelling in New York City. In terms of rehabilitation training, the
Center for Psychiatric Rehabilitation has identified more than 70 practitioner skills that facilitate client participation in a process of achieving success and satisfaction in environments of choice (Anthony,
Cohen and Farkas 1990). Rehabilitation specialists received training
in setting an overall rehabilitation goal, making a functional assessment, direct skills teaching, and case management. They were also
taught the outreach, engagement, survival assessment, and crisis intervention skills that are specific to working with a population of
individuals who are homeless and psychiatrically disabled. In addition to training by the Boston University staff, experts from through-

out the New York City services system trained staff in many of the site-specific issues.

Staff Supervision

Supervision was provided by the on-site director with weekly consultation from the Boston University Center for Psychiatric Rehabilitation. Cases were regularly reviewed to monitor the progress of each program member and to provide feedback to each rehabilitation specialist about the application of skills in specific situations. Peer supervision groups were also initiated to give the rehabilitation specialists the opportunity to learn from each other and to develop creative strategies to deal with difficult skill utilization issues. Program members were interviewed regularly to provide input about how the program was meeting their needs. This feedback was incorporated into the process of supervision and continued program development.

OPERATING THE PROGRAM

While clarification of program mission and values and staff selection and training characterized the early development of the program, its ongoing operation provided many challenges. These challenges involve integrating into and accessing the existing service system, continuing to define and understand the concept of choice particularly in relation to substance use, and developing strategies for involving individuals in long-term community relationships.

Integrating the Program into the New York City Service System

As part of training, staff visited New York City providers to familiarize them with our program and to learn from them about the issues of working in New York City. We also wished to foster collaborative relationships with these providers, to help identify eligible participants, and in the later stages of the research, to locate clients who remained on the street.

We had difficulty enlisting the assistance of some providers. As newcomers, the enthusiasm of our team may have caused us to overemphasize the differences between our approach and those of the existing programs. Our emphasis on the novelty of our approach, our National Institute of Mental Health (NIMH) funding, and the use of the standard treatment system as a control probably heightened competition and distrust. We did not adequately anticipate the reactions of experienced providers. In retrospect, the initiation and integration into the existing system may have been more effective with a humbler and more understated approach. Given our initial presentation and the intrinsically competitive structure of our project, many providers were gracious in accepting us into their community. In addition to problems with other service providers, we also experienced problems with neighborhood resistance to starting another mental health program. Several meetings with representatives from the community board, the State Office of Mental Health, the landlord, and one of the co-investigators were held where we assured the safe and effective operation of the program.

From the Street to the Community: A Developmental Framework for the Application of the Choices Paradigm

During the initial phase of the program, the rehabilitation specialists focused on engaging the client into the program. The client determined the pace and manner of engagement. The program was presented as being flexible and low demand, with only minimum requirements pertaining to everyone's safety. The specialists described the program as a place where people could obtain a wide range of services, from acquiring a bed for the night, clothing, or food to obtaining assistance with the development of a full rehabilitation plan. The specialist was careful not to promise more than could be immediately delivered since the time frame for obtaining services from other agencies was unpredictable.

A subtle and important shift occurred as members became increasingly engaged in the choice-driven program. As the program matured and relationships developed, members were willing to sacrifice some aspects of their personal freedom to obtain desired resources or to participate in community activities. Members decided if and when to make these sacrifices of their personal autonomy in the context of their developing relationship with the program and the desirability of the resource. If the Choices program was to serve its challenging clientele successfully, its evolving normative structure needed to have the flexibility to allow for members' autonomy and self-expression while providing them with shelter, safety, and a sense of belonging.

Collaboration Between Staff and Members

Since the program emphasized a client-directed approach, staff characteristics and their relationships with members were key. In addition to formal training that addressed empathy and connection with the client, we chose staff with backgrounds that were similar to clients in many important respects. Most of the professional and paraprofessional staff represented ethnic and racial minority groups like those of the members. Staff who formerly received mental health services, were homeless, or had problems with alcohol and substance abuse were hired to increase the identification between the members and the staff. The entire respite staff and one-third of the rehabilitation specialists were representatives of one of these groups.

We hypothesized that having a staff with these experiences would be effective for several reasons. Having a combination of professional and recipient staff increased the empathic response in staff-member relationships beyond that found with more traditional staffing patterns, which can be hierarchical or coercive. Staff who have significantly recovered were role models for clients. Direct experience with recovery and/or the mental health system increased sensitivity to the struggles that must be overcome in coping with ongoing psychological problems, adhering to medication regimens, and dealing with power differentials in most therapeutic relationships. Consumer staff were sensitive to members' rights and empowerment.

The use of individuals in recovery who were formerly homeless also presented some difficulties. Former recipients sometimes required supervision in the management of boundaries between staff and members as well as support in their own professional development. Many of the respite staff had spotty work histories and a few experienced problems with attendance that led to large overtime expenses in the program's initial stages. Additionally, several of the respite staff continued to experience problems with alcohol or substances that contributed to their unreliability. Since some staff were struggling with their own recovery, the program attempted to exercise tolerance and compassion on an ongoing basis. This included permitting flexible work schedules and assisting staff to get treatment when they "slipped." The issues and dynamics in managing the program in this manner paralleled the process of working with members to maintain a community that is fair to each individual and still provides enough structure to allow for effective program operation. While we experienced significant paraprofessional turnover in the early phases of the research, we ultimately developed an outstanding paraprofessional staff who were integral to the engagement of members and were essential for successfully operating the program.

In addition to using staff background and experience as an engagement and empowerment strategy, program decision making was also designed to empower members. Initially, decisions regarding program implementation, expenditure of program funds, and the hiring of staff were exclusively the responsibility of the principal investigators and their staff. As members were recruited into the program, their input was incorporated into most decisions regarding program operation. The Center's hours of operation, coordination of shelter beds, and other decisions concerning program management were made jointly by staff and members during the community meeting. Member collaboration also included decisions over program policy and procedure, use of certain grant funds, and relationships with the landlord and the community board. The members eventually formed a Members Council that met on a weekly basis where members voiced their concerns and raised issues to be addressed.

Negotiation and Problem Solving with Individuals Who are Abusing Substances

A constant source of tension between staff, members, and the program model involved the issue of substance abuse. If a member was known to be abusing and/or addicted to drugs or alcohol, the implications of many programmatic decisions differed from those

for individuals who did not abuse substances. Many questions
emerged related to the non-contingent provision of resources
to individuals with addictions and to the management of their
demands on the program when they were intoxicated or in withdrawal. Was giving these individuals food, shelter, and modest cash
subsidies enabling them to spend all of their discretionary funds on
drugs? Were these resources keeping the individual from "bottom-
ing out" and confronting addiction? Should individuals be able to
access their resources whenever they choose, even if the expenditure of cash endangers their ability to meet their monthly housing
obligations? We were unable to arrive at a programmatic resolution
to these questions or to clearly define the boundaries between
honoring individual choice and fostering enablement.

We found that persons addicted to drugs or alcohol made enormous demands on other members and staff, including pleas for both
emotional and instrumental support. If their needs were not met, it
was not uncommon for conversations to escalate to confrontations.
Continual disagreements regarding meeting needs and allocating
resources frustrated the rehabilitation process.

While we did not reach an optimal solution to this dilemma, we
did develop two strategies to help staff manage the ongoing problems with substance abuse and remain consistent with the program
philosophy. The first involved concerted effort at frequent and open
communication among staff regarding the strategy for managing
clients in substance abuse related crisis, thus keeping everyone
aware of the rapidly changing demands of the member and avoid-
ing staff entanglements and contradictions in strategy.

The second strategy involved the use of written contracts between
staff and members. By using contracts that are negotiated when the
member is *not* in crisis and that contain simple and specific language
regarding how the member wishes to be treated in a crisis, the member and staff can refer to their joint understandings in times of crisis.
These points of consensus are likely to become confused when the
member is in a drug-induced state – either high or in withdrawal. The
contract may preserve the member's dignity and sense of control
since it is his/her wishes that guide program behavior.

Since enrollment in the program was not contingent upon being
sober or upon negotiating the contract, it was not used to force individuals into treatment, money management, etc. In rare instances
where members became violent when intoxicated or where, in the
context of a well-established relationship between Choices and the
member, the member was clearly using the program as a "crash
pad" between binges, participation in some aspects of the program
(attending the day center, use of respite beds) was made contingent
upon development of and adherence to a contract.

New York City Specialty Housing: Access Problems and Solutions

One of the most frustrating experiences in developing the experimental program was the process of getting housing. While the City

and the State were involved in an energetic program to designate nearly 5,000 units of specialty housing for persons with mental illness who were homeless, the increased supply of this housing stock did not guarantee access, especially for the relatively more disaffiliated segment of the population that we were serving. Barriers to access involved both client choice and provider rejection of undesirable tenants.

Although rules were often unwritten and subtly expressed, many providers had numerous, rigid criteria for identifying acceptable tenants. These included expectations that persons would readily admit that they were mentally ill, that they would be consistent in taking psychotropic medications and participating in treatment, and that they would follow rules about overnight guests and sobriety, among others. Most SRO hotels required the member to pay two-thirds of his or her Supplemental Security Income (SSI) check for rent, for rooms that ranged in size from 90 to 120 square feet. To complete the eligibility process to apply for specialty housing, individuals had to be interviewed by a psychiatrist, have a psychosocial summary written, and, if approved, participate in interviews with the housing program's clinical and administrative staff. Consistent with State regulation, some State-licensed housing providers required a physical examination.

One member articulated the sentiment of many by saying, "When people want a place to live they want to meet with a landlord, not a psychiatrist." Many Choices members did not wish to participate in the application process given the modest reward of an SRO room with many restrictions. Some members refused to label themselves as mentally ill. Additionally, sacrificing nearly all of their discretionary income for rent was a difficult transition for many members, especially in light of their full access to church shelter beds. Given these alternatives, many members chose to remain in the respite housing.

Not only were members rejecting housing providers, most providers were extremely hesitant to accept our applicants. Exclusionary rules concerning sobriety and failure to complete a transitional program were the two major reasons for rejection. Additionally, many of the residential programs were in a "rent-up" phase in which their operating costs were subsidized by either the City or the State. This subsidy, along with strong tenants' rights laws in the City that made it very difficult to evict problem tenants, encouraged landlords to avoid risks with our members.

Programmatically, we had reached a disturbing impasse. We had created a safe and comfortable environment for the members who had been successfully engaged into the program. The housing alternatives available, however, were somewhat unappealing to our members, who, in turn, were generally unappealing to the housing providers. The limited capacity of our respite program was restricting our ability to bring new members from the streets, which was a critical part of our program mission. The program was in gridlock.

We spent several months trying to find a solution to this predicament. Our strategy involved working with the members, continuing to work with housing providers, and seeking housing providers who might be convinced to work with our group. Additionally, we employed a psychiatrist to drop by the program one afternoon a week and slowly develop relationships with the members. The psychiatric component of the evaluation could then be completed and the members' psychiatric needs addressed more generally.

Our strategy for working directly with the members involved improving their overall appeal to landlords. Consultants suggested that we personalize the application of each member by including a nice photograph, writing a long letter emphasizing the gains the member had made, how likeable he/she was, etc. Other advisors urged us to train clients to be more effective during interviews by teaching them not to ask too many questions, not to talk about alcohol or substance abuse, or not to focus on procedures for having overnight guests. Essentially, the messages were always the same: Just try to fit in. We, therefore, began a series of skills training interventions to make our clients more successful in the landlord interview process.

We provided tours of the homeless specialty housing both to educate the members regarding the choices that were available within this housing system and to educate staff regarding the various requirements of providers and the properties that they had available. This continued exposure both helped clients develop a context within which to evaluate any given housing setting and exposed our program to these providers. It was our impression that this familiarity and growing acceptance into the general provider community in the City significantly improved our ability to work within this network.

A major breakthrough in the housing placement bottleneck was achieved when we identified a housing provider who agreed to consider our members on the condition that Choices guaranteed to provide needed, ongoing support to the members after they were housed. Importantly, this provider operated a supported housing program that was using State rent subsidies to access general market housing (i.e., scattered-site apartments). The provider, therefore, was not the landlord, but served as a broker between landlords and tenants and guaranteed rent to the landlords. With this provider, we obtained apartments that members found more desirable than serviced SRO hotel rooms. The availability of this housing broke the program gridlock.

As a follow-up to identifying and working with this provider, a new supported housing program called Pathways to Housing, Inc., was created with one of our co-principal investigators (S.T.) taking responsibility for organizing the new corporation. With this program we were able to augment the support available to members of Choices (as well as others) and to operate our own scatter-site supported apartment program. Typically, supported apartment programs served graduates of community residences or supported SROs. However, after some advocacy and lobbying on our part, Pathways obtained the contract to provide these services and housing settings to the street population.

Keeping the Housing: Ongoing Problems With Support and Rehabilitation

After successfully obtaining housing for a substantial number of the Choices members, we began to confront the issue of helping individuals to keep their housing. Problems adjusting to housing exaggerated problems with alcohol and substance abuse. We continued to seek more effective ways to support members in their rehabilitation while keeping them in their housing settings.

People with substance abuse problems were the most difficult to support because of the intensity of their needs. They often invited others, who used crack cocaine, into their apartments and sometimes through these associations became involved in selling cocaine or in carrying out other illegal activities to obtain crack. Similarly, they were likely to be victimized in their apartments. When individuals were actively using crack, they often were not interested in working with or being seen by their rehabilitation specialists and this reduced the contact with a support person at a time when it was needed the most. As we discussed earlier, we used various strategies to encourage these individuals to enter treatment. We sponsored AA and NA meetings at the Center and held groups that addressed issues of substance and alcohol abuse. We were never satisfied that we had developed a generally effective strategy.

A related problem involved the lack of meaningful daytime activities for most members. Other than occasional work, nearly all of the experimental subjects (96.7 %) were unemployed and generally not involved in meaningful productive activities. Some individuals assumed volunteer roles at the program as a way of keeping busy and contributing to the Choices community. Others participated in a Center-sponsored volunteer program to distribute clothes in the neighborhood. However, most were not interested in these activities and sought some form of paid employment. Vocational opportunities would have been very helpful in keeping individuals housed.

Although the Center was available to members once they became housed, many of the housing units were not in the neighborhood. It therefore became difficult for members to remain in contact with the Choices community. Housing located in poor neighborhoods increased the likelihood that members would become involved with the drug culture. When alcohol and drugs were not a problem, social isolation diminished the individual's quality of life and may have substantially decreased the value of the housing to the individual.

We developed supportive activities to stay in touch with individuals who were housed and to assist them to develop relationships in their communities. We encouraged them to visit the Center and sponsored monthly alumni dinners. Occasionally individuals who were housed used the respite beds to spend time with their friends who had not yet become housed. Members were invited by the Pathways to Housing staff to a weekly movie night with other tenants. Helping members to maintain contact with the Choices community or to integrate into their new communities was an ongoing challenge to the program. If the program is to prove successful in the long term, it must successfully confront these ongoing issues.

THE RESEARCH PROGRAM INTERFACE

Conducting the project as a research demonstration had several effects on the program operation. While we believe that these were generally positive, they also were the source of tension between the research and program staff. The principal areas in which the research affected the program involved the clarity of program values that resulted from continual review of the research hypotheses, the tensions of constant scrutiny, the use of the research information systems, and the freedom to innovate and fail derived from program's experimental nature.

Clarity of Program Mission

Perhaps the most far-ranging impact of operating the project as a research demonstration was on the clarity of program mission, values, approaches, and outcomes. Designing a successful research demonstration required that we clearly articulate the rationale for our approach and the key hypotheses of the study. The rationale related both to the structure and function of the program and emphasized fostering client choice, being responsible for a designated group of experimental clients, and maintaining the continuity of relationships with the clients. Our hypotheses focused on improving client outcomes particularly in the areas of housing status and quality of life. Both the rationale and hypotheses had consistent effects on the operation of the program.

As an organizing principle, choice was a constant source of discussion among the program staff. To the degree to which members failed as a result of their choices (e.g., failed to obtain housing because they wouldn't attempt to stop using substances), staff began to doubt the value of the choice paradigm. Rather than the model drifting away from a client-driven to a staff-driven approach, however, the continual focus on the study rationale required the staff and members to innovate, accommodate their differences, and reconceptualize the meaning of choice as the program evolved. The discussion and management of the program, therefore, consistently focused on this central value giving continuity and stability to the program model.

Continuity and stability were also enhanced through the single point of responsibility implicit in the experimental design and the focus on program outcomes. These factors prohibited staff from withdrawing services from particularly difficult individuals. This was challenging – especially for the few members who exhibited violent or threatening behavior. Clear guidelines, primarily related to safety, guided the staff's interactions with threatening or violent individuals. Without the single point of responsibility and accountability that were part of the experiment, we suspect that these members would have been terminated from the program.

This "no reject" policy also had powerful negotiating potential that was quickly and astutely understood by the members. Members were empowered because, unlike other programs from which they had been banned, Choices would maintain contact with them at all costs. Differences of opinion between members and staff had to be resolved for the staff to succeed. The clients' success and the staffs' effectiveness were inextricably commingled. This arrangement served to make staff and clients more accepting of one another and more likely to diligently resolve their differences.

The focus on outcomes helped direct program activities. Within the constraints of client choice and the program model, we continually focused on improving client housing status and quality of life. Since these targets were operationalized quantitatively, the staff knew the degree to which they were achieving the major program outcomes, which importantly assisted them in organizing their work.

It is our impression from other programs that we have operated or evaluated that this clarity in program mission, values, approaches, and outcomes is often missing. We feel that the successful implementation of the program is directly attributable to the structure and methods of the research demonstration and the specificity of the psychiatric rehabilitation philosophy and technology.

Constant Scrutiny

To successfully follow this homeless sample, interviewers and qualitative researchers maintained close contact and developed ongoing relationships with the research participants. When members became dissatisfied with the services that they were receiving at Choices, they sometimes felt as though the interviewers had misled them. This role confusion for the interviewers, which involved having to represent the program in the engagement process while independently assessing its outcomes, strained relationships between the interviewers and both the members and program staff. Interviewers' complaints about the program angered program staff who felt that the interviewers had only partial information about a member's situation. Relatedly, a qualitative researcher, who was stationed at the program 20 hours per week and who became very involved with the members, was seen as intrusive and as an advocate.

We addressed these tensions by increasing the number of interactions between interviewers and rehabilitation staff in both formal and informal contexts and by continually stressing the shared purpose of their work. We attempted to reconceptualize criticism as valuable program feedback that could be used to change program operations. We also focused on the boundary issues researchers confront as they attempt to clarify differences between their roles as researchers and as individuals concerned with the welfare of participants in their study. These strategies seem to have been moderately successful in reducing the ongoing tension among the staff and in maintaining the objectivity of the research staff – a difficult challenge given the intensity of the relationships established over two years of interactions.

Research Information System

Our continuous monitoring of the program staff activities and the production of routine reports of program outcomes positively impacted the program. Quantifying the rate at which clients were engaged in the program and the rate at which they were being housed allowed us to provide bi-weekly feedback to the program on its success and to critically evaluate our strategies for improving program performance. Interestingly, in a program with significant data collection requirements, Choices staff independently developed a client status form that was used for monitoring members' progress. They regularly completed this form without oversight. Routine quantitative information from the research, therefore, was valued and incorporated into the management of the program.

Freedom to Innovate and Fail

The final impact of administering the program as a research demonstration was a freedom to innovate and to fail. Particularly in light of the ongoing evaluation of program performance, we realized the importance of creating an "experimenting" culture. We stressed that our primary mission was to test the experimental propositions in a very challenging environment. Failure to accomplish specific goals for members or overall program goals were considered learning opportunities – ones in which we would attempt to abstract the principles or techniques that seemed inappropriate. This lessened the evaluation anxiety and freed the staff to innovate and reflect on their actions. It is perhaps the spirit of experimentation, when coupled with a clarity of purpose, systematic feedback regarding the program outcomes, and the processes which either produced or frustrated these outcomes that best expresses the benefits of developing a program as a research demonstration.

EARLY FINDINGS

We have completed some analyses of both the qualitative and quantitative data. While we will not provide any detail regarding these analyses here, we will highlight some of the major findings. These relate to the nature of the experimental program and of the standard treatment control and to the outcome results. A more complete presentation of these findings is included in a paper by Shern, Lovell, Tsemberis *et al.* 1994.

Nature of the Experimental Program and Standard Treatment

We have completed three sub-studies to document the program intervention and to contrast it with the standard treatment control. The first involved the use of concept mapping techniques (Trochim 1989) to assess the degree to which we successfully transferred the program model from the BU Center for Psychiatric Rehabilitation to the Choices program in New York City (see Shern, Trochim, and LaComb 1995).

In brief, the results from this study indicate that the model was successfully transferred. Substantial overlap was found in the concepts that characterize the Choices program and those identified as key by the BU staff. A correlation of .76 was found between the similarity matrices for BU and Choices while the multidimensional scaling of these matrices produced maps with a correlation of .37. Both correlations are significant. These quantitative indicators of similarity and the literal interpretation of the maps indicate successful transfer of the model. Some interesting adaptations occurred in transferring the models. Most importantly, while the BU staff conceptualized case management and rehabilitation as an integrated set of activities, the Choices staff conceptualized them as distinct. Case management related more closely to acquiring housing and meeting basic needs for the Choices staff than it did for the BU staff.

In the second study, Lovell and Cohn (in press) used a variety of qualitative research techniques to investigate the degree to which the concept of client direction and choice characterized the experimental intervention. Results generally indicate that these concepts were central operating principles of the program. Although clients were initially incredulous regarding the degree to which their choices would be paramount in designing a rehabilitation program, over time a culture evolved in the program that supported the importance of choice and client direction in all aspects of the program. This culture led generally to more egalitarian relationships between staff and clients than might typically be the case.

The third sub-study involved documenting the services available to the control subjects in the standard treatment environment. As with both of the earlier studies, the results of this study are complex and are available in a paper by Lovell, Richmond, and Shern (1993). The major findings indicate that substantial overlap existed between the services that were generally available in the standard treatment condition and those offered by the Choices program. However, standard treatment programs often were missing two components of psychiatric rehabilitation: client advocacy and an emphasis on client rights. Most standard treatment programs did not have an identified group of clients whom they were obligated to serve. Semi-structured interviews with the care providers and control subjects suggested that the control programs generally had normatively defined goals that were based on a priori notions of acceptable behaviors rather than an idiographic emphasis on client definition of needs and goals.

The evaluation of the standard treatment condition when combined with the Lovell and Cohn (in press) study generally confirms
our expectations regarding the differences between standard treatment and the experimental program. While both offer a largely
overlapping array of services, the organization of services and their
overall orientation differ in the ways that we hypothesized to be
important for engaging and serving this population.

EARLY OUTCOME RESULTS

Analysis of the outcome and client status variables generally favor
the experimental program. In terms of client status variables, individuals in the experimental program report a significantly greater
reduction in problems with symptoms than control group members.
No significant between-group differences are noted for measures of
self-esteem or mastery, while individuals in the experimental group
report rates of goal attainment that are double those of control
group subjects.

Individuals assigned to the experimental program had more
favorable housing outcomes than control subjects. Over the 24-month
follow-up interval, experimental group members experienced a 57%
reduction in their time spent on the streets as opposed to a 30%
reduction for the control group. Similarly, the experimental group
had an increase in time spent in shelters and long-term community
housing settings by 23% and 22%, respectively, while the control
group showed almost no increase in shelter use (up only 3% from
baseline) and an 11% increase in time spent in community residential
settings. While the between-group differences for these three settings
attain conventional levels of statistical significance ($p < .01$), no
between-group differences were obtained for time spent in institutions (e.g., hospitals, jails).

The two groups also are significantly different in their 24-month
change scores for six of the seven subjective quality of life scales
from the Lehman (1988) measure. Relative to the control group
members, members of the experimental group report a 0.6 standard
deviation improvement in their overall quality of life and improve-
ments that average 0.46 standard deviation units for each of the
other five quality of life areas: leisure (.35), financial (.65), safety
(.44), health (.43), and family (.46). Only satisfaction with social relationships did not attain statistical significance ($p = .056$) but the
between-group differences did favor the experimental condition.

DISCUSSION AND IMPLICATIONS

This study was purposely designed to test several important
hypotheses regarding public policies and practices for serving difficult and disaffiliated populations. Given the relative success of the
Choices program in meeting client and social needs and the under-

standing of the process that has emerged from the careful study of this program, we have identified four areas of policy and practice for which the research may be particularly relevant.

Access

Individuals who are street dwelling and who have psychiatric disabilities report difficulty gaining access to the human service system; we hypothesized that both structural and functional components of the system contribute to this difficulty. The clients' reports of their experiences with standard mental health programming, our difficulty in obtaining specialty housing, and our study of the standard treatment environment all supported these hypotheses regarding system barriers.

These clients had rejected and been rejected by the standard treatment approaches. Perhaps most fundamentally, their mutual rejection relates to the expectations of many standard treatment providers regarding client conformity to social norms. Rather than starting with a client's conception of his/her situation and needs, some providers reject the client as "not ready" for a program if the client's perceived needs and strategies differ from those of the provider. Programs seek clients whom they feel will benefit from their services, meaning that clients who are most disaffiliated and needy may go unserved.

By explicitly orienting the program around client choice and direction, we seem to have addressed this initial disjuncture between the member and the program. Services began wherever the member preferred. Then, through an evolving connection between the client and the program, we sought to meet each client's self-identified goals. Given the resource constraints of the program, the resulting need to obtain services from the external environment, as well as the evolving needs of the Choices community itself, the concept of choice changed as individuals participated in the program. Nonetheless, this strong client-centered orientation clearly distinguished the Choices program from standard treatment and was reported by members in the qualitative study to be a defining characteristic of the program's appeal. Therefore, the client-centered orientation may importantly underlie the successful engagement of clients in the experimental group and the differential positive outcomes for the experimental group.

Another important program feature that improved access involved hiring staff who represent the ethnic, cultural, and experiential characteristics of the clients. Employing consumers has proven to be an invaluable asset of our program.

From a public policy and practice perspective, barriers to access which are related to program expectations for successful participation should be carefully examined. Clients should be engaged on their terms, their choices and goals should be honored and the consequences of their choices observed before excluding them from participation.

A related structural barrier involves the lack of a single point of responsibility for identified clients – particularly the most difficult to serve. When programs are not held responsible for identified individuals, they are able to reject individuals who they believe are not ready for their programs. Under such circumstances, the client's ability to negotiate with the program is substantially reduced. The power dynamics change, however, if the program must serve pre-identified individuals and be held responsible for their outcomes. For the most needy clients who have traditionally been rejected by the human service system, this structural element seems to be key.

Outcome Monitoring from Multiple Perspectives

Programs must make quantitative assessments of their success in meeting client goals. Funding agencies cannot hold programs accountable without outcome measures. Program self-study and change in intervention strategy also require information on program outcomes. We found that constant focus on the major intended outcomes of the project when coupled with information about staff behavior was very helpful in evaluating differing strategies for meeting client needs.

It is important that outcomes be designed for each intended component of the program model (e.g., engagement, leaving the street, entitlements, housing, quality of life), that they be simple to measure and meaningful to the staff, and that they be simultaneously measured throughout the duration of the project as long as they are relevant. Ideally, the relationship between differing patterns of staff behavior and client outcomes could be explored quantitatively. Without the systematic assessment and examination of outcomes, it is literally impossible to determine if policy changes regarding access and accountability are effectively addressing client needs.

Reimbursement Mechanisms

Program reimbursement should parallel program goals. Often, reimbursement is based exclusively on the volume of services that are provided. This design may emphasize the creation of dependency between the program and the client since revenues are maximized when individuals receive more services and stay longer in the program. Similarly, without client assignment, individuals are likely to be selected for a program when they desire the program's services and are willing to receive a large volume of them. While it is important to be able to summarize the type and frequency of services provided, these data are only informative in light of the outcomes that the program is producing. Reimbursing for outcomes is a much preferred policy alternative.

Problems of Alcohol and Other Substance Abuse

As we noted throughout this chapter, the complications represented by alcohol and substance abuse are enormous. While we feel that it is clearly inappropriate to bar individuals from housing based upon the presence of addictions, we readily admit that keeping individuals with addictions in housing is much more difficult than we anticipated. Programs designed to serve individuals with mental illness who are homeless must anticipate that the majority of these individuals will also have problems with alcohol and substance abuse and plan for supportive and treatment services. These services can either be provided directly or obtained from other providers. From a public policy perspective, any system barrier to effective integration of alcohol and substance abuse services should be eliminated – this is particularly important for meeting the unique needs of this population group. Finally, it is our impression that much work remains to be completed in developing and evaluating effective technologies and programs for individuals with these co-morbidities.

SUMMARY

While our experiences implementing and studying this program indicate that successfully engaging and assisting street dwelling individuals who have psychiatric disabilities is very difficult, our data clearly indicate that the problems of this population can be addressed. A responsive program grounded in psychiatric rehabilitation philosophy and technology that honors the client perspective, provides a meaningful and accessible community for its members, advocates for clients' needs in the larger services community, and provides the supports and skills training necessary to assist clients in meeting their objectives can serve even the most disaffiliated individuals. It is our hope that this intensive study of this particular client group will suggest changes in policy and practice that may improve the access to services for other, similarly situated persons and, ultimately, the trajectory of their reintegration and recovery.

REFERENCES

Anthony, W.A., Cohen, M.R. & Farkas, M. (1990). *Psychiatric rehabilitation.* Boston: Boston University Center for Psychiatric Rehabilitation.

Barrow, S.M. (1988). *Delivery of services to homeless mentally ill clients: Engagement, direct service and intensive case management at five CSS programs.* Unpublished manuscript.

Cohen, M., Danley, K. & Nemec, P. (1985). *Training technology: Direct skills teaching.* Boston: Boston University Center for Psychiatric Rehabilitation.

Cohen, M., Farkas, M. & Cohen, B. (1986). *Training technology: Functional assessment.* Boston: Boston University Center for Psychiatric Rehabilitation.

Cohen, M., Farkas, M. & Cohen, B. (1992). *Training technology: Assessing readiness for rehabilitation.* Boston: Boston University Center for Psychiatric Rehabilitation.

Cohen, M., Farkas, M., Cohen, B. & Unger, K. (1990). *Training technology: Getting overall rehabilitation goals.* Boston: Boston University Center for Psychiatric Rehabilitation.

Cohen, M. & Forbess, R. (1993). *Training technology: Developing readiness for rehabilitation.* Boston: Boston University Center for Psychiatric Rehabilitation.

Cohen, M., Nemec, P., Farkas, M. & Forbess, R. (1988). *Training technology: Person-oriented case management.* Boston: Boston University Center for Psychiatric Rehabilitation.

Cohen, N.L., Putnam, J.F. & Sullivan, A.M. (1984). The mentally ill homeless: Isolation and adaptation. *Hospital and Community Psychiatry* 35: 922–924.

Cohen, N.L. & Tsemberis, S. (1991). Emergency psychiatric intervention on the street. *New Directions for Mental Health Services* 52:3–16.

Dion, G.L. & Anthony, W.A. (1987). Research in psychiatric rehabilitation: A review of experimental and quasi-experimental studies. *Rehabilitation Counseling Bulletin* 30:177–203.

Freddolino, P.P. & Moxley, D.P. (1992). Clinical care update: Refining an advocacy model for homeless people coping with psychiatric disabilities. *Community Mental Health Journal* 28(4):337–352.

Lehman, A.F. (1988). Quality of life interview for the chronically mentally ill. *Evaluation and Program Planning* 11(1):51–62.

Lovell, A.M. & Cohn, S. (in press). The elaboration of choice in a program for homeless persons labeled psychiatrically disabled. *Human Organization.*

Lovell, A.M., Richmond, L. & Shern, D.L. (1993). *Standard treatment for the homeless mentally ill.* In preparation.

Plapinger, J.D. (1988). *Program service goals: Service needs, service feasibility, and obstacles to providing services to the mentally ill homeless.* Unpublished manuscript.

Shern, D.L. (1993). *Housing mentally ill street people: A rehab approach.* (NIMH Grant Proposal). Albany: New York State Office of Mental Health, Bureau of Evaluation and Services Research.

Shern, D.L. (1990). *Housing mentally ill street people: A rehab approach.* (NIMH Grant Proposal R18 MH48215). Albany: New York State Office of Mental Health, Bureau of Evaluation and Services Research.

Shern, D.L., Surles, R.C. & Waizer, J. (1989). Designing community treatment systems for the most seriously mentally ill: A state administrative perspective. *Journal of Social Issues* 45:105–117.

Shern, D.L., Trochim, W.M. & LaComb, C. (1995). The use of concept mapping for assessing fidelity of model transfer: An example from psychiatric rehabilitation. *Evaluation and Program Planning* 18(2):143–153.

Shern, D.L., Lovell, A.M., Tsemberis, S., LaComb, C.A., Anthony, W., Richmond, L., Winarski, J. & Cohen, M. (1994). Rehabilitation of homeless street dwelling individuals with mental illness. *Proceedings of the Fourth Conference on State Mental Health Agency Services Research.* Alexandria, VA: National Association of State Mental Health Program Directors Research Institute.

Struening, E.L. (1986). *A study of residents of the New York City shelter system.* An unpublished report prepared for the Department of Mental Health,

Mental Retardation and Alcoholism Services. New York: New York State Psychiatric Institute.

Susser, E., Goldfinger, S. & White, A. (1990). Some clinical approaches to the homeless mentally ill. *Community Mental Health Journal* 26(5):463–480.

Tessler, R.C. & Dennis, D.L. (1989). A synthesis of NIMH-funded research concerning persons who are homeless and mentally ill. Unpublished manuscript.

Tsemberis, S., Cohen, N.L. & Jones, R. (1993). Conducting emergency psychiatric evaluations on the street. In S. Katz, D. Nardacci, & A. Sabatini (Eds.), Intensive treatment of the homeless mentally ill. Washington, DC: American Psychiatric Press.

NOTE

This research was supported by a grant from the National Institute of Mental Health and the Center for Mental Health Services (MH-48215). Portions of this paper were abstracted from a research proposal submitted to the National Institute of Mental Health (Shern 1993) and from *Proceedings of the Fourth Annual Research Conference of the National Association of State Mental Health Program Directors Research Institute, 1994.*

8

Transitional vs. Permanent Housing: Lessons From a Research Plan That Did Not Work Out as Planned

JANET FORD, ROBERT L. OBERMEYER,
JAMES E. HEALY, BEVERLY GENTRY,
DONALD ROHNER and JAMES R. HILLARD

This chapter reports on a project that did not receive continuing funding for the proposed third year of operation. The Cincinnati Project operated for three years: from January 1, 1991 through December 31, 1993. It received funding for two of the proposed years: September 30, 1990 through August 31, 1992. Funding was discontinued at the recommendation of the site visit team from the National Institute of Mental Health (NIMH), following their visit to and review of the Cincinnati Project in April, 1992. The site visit team stated that the decision to terminate funding was based on two research implementation issues: 1) recruitment of clients to the project programs was well behind the proposed and projected figures; and 2) random assignment of clients and baseline data collection procedures were determined to be unscientific and inconsistent with the other study sites, although they followed the protocol established in the original project proposal.

Despite the fact that the project completed a third year of operation with funds carried over from the first and second years of the grant, the failure of the project to meet its projected figures and to complete the proposed research was upsetting and embarrassing to the Cincinnati Project administrators at the Hamilton County Community Mental Health Board (HCCMHB). Some of the problems that contributed to the project's lack of success were unavoidable; others probably could have been prevented or their consequences minimized with better planning and administration. It is hoped that the process of reviewing our errors with proverbial 20–20 hindsight will be useful to future researchers. Perhaps others can benefit from the experience.

BACKGROUND

The proposed research was originally suggested by the Director of Housing and Residential Services at the HCCMHB. As a planner and administrator of residential services for persons with severe mental illness in the county, he was interested in conducting a structured, scientific comparison of transitional versus permanent housing models of service. The superiority of transitional vs. permanent housing programs for persons with severe mental illness was a question that had frequently been debated by service planners and funding bodies. Carling and Ridgeway (1989) identified two of "the most critical issues in the field" of psychiatric rehabilitation as: 1) the "extent to which housing needs should be met in 'residential facilities', that is, discrete residential programs, or in normal housing linked to services"; and 2) "whether 'transitions' should necessarily, or even typically, involve changing one's housing arrangement"(p. 69). They suggested that long-term support to consumers in a range of permanent housing settings, as opposed to the "transitional models that now predominate in this field" (p. 70) were needed. The housing philosophies espoused by the psychiatric rehabilitation model are drawn from and reflect the normalization and community support systems models of mental health treatment (Turner & Ten-Hoor, 1978; Carling, 1984) which promote the philosophy that "skills should be taught in the actual location where they will be used" rather than trying to transfer skills learned in a transitional setting to the long-term housing situation (Carling & Ridgeway, 1989, p. 71).

At the time the project proposal was being developed, the Ohio Department of Mental Health (ODMH) was promoting the psychosocial rehabilitation model and a policy that permanent housing should be provided as a basic community support for mentally ill persons in need of residences. The "housing as housing" policy was that community mental health services should be provided in the client's normal or natural community environment, not in transitional residential programs (Ohio Department of Mental Health, 1988).

On the other side, arguments could be found endorsing transitional housing programs to serve the homeless mentally ill, who, in contrast to other persons with mental illness, are more mobile, disaffiliated, and resistant to traditional treatment approaches (Appleby, Slagg & Desai, 1982; Bachrach, 1982; Goldfinger & Chafetz, 1984; & Lamb, 1984). Levine (1984) suggested that the homeless mentally ill frequently "need the flexibility, informality, and non-invasiveness" of transitional arrangements to move toward longer periods of more stable residence (p. 196). She also pointed out that "because of the nature of their mental disabilities and the paucity of appropriate residential options, it is often impossible to make perma-

nent living arrangements for the homeless mentally ill during the
short stay permitted in an emergency shelter" (p. 190). Baxter and
Hopper (1984) suggested that transitional accommodations might
provide a needed level of shelter between emergency shelter and permanent housing, where homeless clients' differentiated needs would
be addressed, necessary entitlements and clinical linkages pursued,
and an individualized permanent housing plan made. The support-
ers of transitional housing advocated its use to complement emergency shelters and to "engage the disengaged" by "providing an
environment in which homeless mentally ill clients can make the
physical and emotional transition from shelter to long-term housing"
(Levine, 1984, p. 196; Stroul, 1988).

Tender Mercies, Inc., using matching funds from the HCCMHB,
had received a McKinney Grant to establish the Step-up Transitional
Housing Program for Homeless Severely Mentally Disabled Adults.
The Step-up Program opened in 1988 with a capacity of 5 beds and
was in the process of expanding to 16 beds. Thus, the HCCMHB's
Housing and Residential Services program was administering programs to support permanent housing options for persons with mental illness under the ODMH "housing as housing" policy, but also
contracting with the Step-up Program to provide *transitional* housing for homeless persons with severe mental illness. Review of the
literature did not locate any studies specifically comparing the
effectiveness of the two types of housing programs. The question
persisted as an issue to be examined in planning residential services
for homeless mentally ill persons.

The Cincinnati project attempted to build on the groundwork
established by previous projects to provide services to homeless
persons with mental illness in Hamilton County. As stated, the transitional program for the project was originally funded in part by a
McKinney Grant. It had been in limited operation for over two years
at the time of the grant proposal and had recently expanded its
building capacity from 5 to 16 beds.

The permanent housing program was developed specifically for
the project but utilized permanent housing options which were
operationally modified for the research project but were already
part of a system of housing units owned, operated, or under contract by the HCCMHB. These units included scattered site apartments, clustered apartments, and single room occupancy (SRO)
units, most of which were funded through subsidies made available
by the Ohio Department of Mental Health's Housing Assistance
program and controlled by the HCCMHB. Under the terms of the
rental agreements, the HCCMHB leased units and sublet them to
program participants.

SUMMARY OF PROJECT PROPOSAL

The Cincinnati Site Project proposal was the first attempt by HCCMHB
personnel to apply directly for a federal research project grant.
This project was intended to compare the efficacy of transitional vs.

permanent housing for homeless mentally ill persons in Hamilton
County, Ohio (Cincinnati). Program participants had to meet the following inclusion criteria: age 18 years or older; with a diagnosis of
psychotic or affective disorders according to DSM-III-R (American
Psychiatric Association, 1987); and homeless, i.e., "lacking a fixed,
regular, and adequate nighttime residence". Persons meeting these
criteria were randomly assigned to either: 1) a transitional program
from which they would "graduate" to permanent housing arrangements or 2) a permanent program which would help them locate
and adjust to non-transitional housing options.

The two programs were to provide equivalent support services
to the project clients. These services included on-site case management, psychiatric treatment, and skills training to prepare clients to
live in permanent housing options. The discharge plans for clients
in both programs were for them to obtain permanent housing and
to progress from their respective programs to community mental
health services, including case management.

The main difference between the two programs was the setting
in which clients obtained the skills training to prepare them for
community living. Clients in the *transitional* program lived in the
program's "group rooming house" setting during their program
stay and then, upon graduation, moved into permanent housing
arrangements in the community. Clients in the *permanent* program
were given the option of remaining in the apartment in which they
had resided during their program stay when, upon graduation, they
were transferred from the program to regular community mental
health services. Since the transitional program had a capacity of
16 beds, the permanent program was also limited to 16 clients at
any given time. Based on the transitional program's historical performance, it was projected that during the 3 year proposed study
period, approximately 60 clients would be served by each program,
for a total of 120 project clients.

The study hypothesis was that the transitional program would be
as effective but more cost-efficient than the permanent program in
helping clients adjust to living in permanent housing. Outcome
measures included clinical status, functional level, quality of life,
housing stability, and use of psychiatric and mental health services.

IMPLEMENTATION

The study grant was awarded in October 1990 and the project start-
up began immediately thereafter in order to be operational for study
participants by January 1991. This start-up date was three months
earlier than proposed, due to the Federal funding schedule. The loss
of three months of anticipated planning and preparation time was
weighed against the loss of the "window of opportunity" to obtain
the funding necessary to launch a project of this type. The opportunity to compare the merits and weaknesses of transitional vs. supported permanent housing options for a multi-problem group of
persons with severe mental illness seemed too great to give up, par-

ticularly since it appeared to be a one-time, "take it or lose it forever" chance. The proposed project seemed to epitomize applied research; an empirical study which would have "real world" applications. This aspect of the proposal was especially appealing to the Cincinnati site project administrators at the HCCMHB.

The first phase of project implementation included 1) hiring of research personnel to conduct the study and 2) the creation of the permanent program: setting up permanent housing options and hiring staff to provide services to the clients. This start-up phase necessitated the cooperative efforts of three separate agencies.

First, the HCCMHB, which initiated the proposal and was administering the overall research project, hired and trained the research associates to collect study data and maintain the project database. The HCCMHB also operated the Housing and Residential Services Program which leased the housing units to be occupied by the permanent program participants. The second agency involved in the project was Tender Mercies, Inc., the agency which already operated the transitional program and was to operate the permanent program and provide case management and independent living skills training to study participants in both programs. The third project agency was Psychiatric Professional Services, Inc. (PPSI), a non-profit corporation affiliated with the University of Cincinnati Department of Psychiatry. PPSI was already providing on-site psychiatric services to Tender Mercies clients, including diagnostic assessments using the Structured Clinical Interview for DSM-III-R (SCID) (Spitzer, Williams & Gibbon, 1986). PPSI contract staff were to do the SCID assessments for prospective study participants.

Administrative Issues

Despite the relatively small size of the project and the fact that the three agencies had a history of working together, project implementation encountered a number of problems, many of which stemmed from organizational changes in Tender Mercies, Inc. Administrative problems could be identified at the two service agencies and at the overall project level.

Overall project level: The HCCMHB was and is primarily an administrative agency which contracts with community mental health service agencies and other service providers to deliver services to clients under its jurisdiction. Services to participants in the research project were not directly administered by the researchers, as the Principal Investigator and research associates were employees of the HCCMHB. The HCCMHB had a contractual agreement with Tender Mercies, Inc., that Tender Mercies staff would a) conduct outreach to homeless shelters and other services where potential study participants could be located and recruited, b) admit participants to randomly assigned housing (either transitional or permanent program) and provide them with case management and independent living skills training, and c) transfer participants from both programs to traditional community mental health services when they were ready to "graduate" from the Tender Mercies programs. The project service providers on the Tender Mercies staff reported to the Executive Director of that agency. The HCCMHB also had a contractual agreement with PPSI to conduct the SCID assessments of potential study participants in order to confirm their psychiatric eligibility for the study.

HCCMHB personnel directly administered a) random assignment of potential study participants to programs, b) collection, management, and analysis of study data, and c) leasing and maintenance of permanent housing options for immediate occupancy by study participants randomly assigned to the permanent program. As part of the overall project administration, representatives from the three project agencies were scheduled to meet on a monthly basis or more frequently to monitor project implementation and to identify and address problems. Attendance at these meetings was inconsistent on the part of the service agency personnel. Both of the agencies were undergoing major changes which were not directly related to the research project, but which had adverse effects upon its implementation.

Tender Mercies, Inc.: This agency was the project keystone. The transitional program was already in operation at this agency and it had a good reputation in the community, particularly with other agencies and programs serving homeless individuals. The agency had undergone major changes in personnel and administration shortly before the project was proposed.

Tender Mercies, Inc., was founded and originally operated by two Catholic priests who were known as long-time community activists and advocates for homeless mentally ill persons in the Cincinnati area. One of the priests was the Executive Director of the agency from the time of its inception until his illness and death shortly before the project was proposed. The other priest served as Associate Executive Director until his transfer to another state shortly before the Executive Director became ill. The agency benefitted greatly from the leadership of its founders: their vision of what the program should be, contacts with other community leaders and service providers, experience in community organization, and ability to attract and delegate responsibilities to capable volunteers and staff.

The project startup coincided with the internal promotion of the director of the transitional program to the position of Executive Director at Tender Mercies. In terms of the research project, this new Executive Director had the responsibility of hiring a new program director, doubling the size of the program staff from approximately 8 to approximately 16 FTE direct service workers, and training all the workers to provide the services according to the project proposal. Had this person remained as program director, the start-up process probably would have been less problematic. The *agency* as a whole still would have been affected by the difficulties of replacing the experienced and charismatic agency founders, but the study *program* might have maintained some stability in its operation. As it was, the Executive Director apparently was overwhelmed by the additional responsibilities and demands of the promotion and lacking the support from both the agency Board of Trustees and the community at large that the previous Executive Director had enjoyed.

Psychiatric Professional Services, Inc.: This agency also experienced administrative changes which affected the project. The psychiatric assessments for the study participants were still conducted by PPSI, but in a different manner than was originally planned. A psychiatrist working with PPSI had established a program for University of Cincinnati psychiatry residents interested in working with community residents with severe mental illnesses. This program had contracted with Tender Mercies, Inc., to serve the agency's clients on site. Psychiatric assessments of potential study participants would have been contracted through this program. While the research project was still in the proposal stage, this psychiatrist left the University of Cincinnati's Department of Psychiatry to take a position in another state. As a result of the psychiatrist's departure, the program for residents was virtually discontinued at Tender Mercies, although PPSI continued to contract for services with Tender Mercies, Inc., and with the HCCMHB to conduct SCID diagnostic assessments. The departure of the enthusiastic and experienced program psychiatrist left another major gap in terms of leadership that might have helped in dealing with some of the problems in coordinating the project effort.

Service Provision Issues

Service provision was adversely affected by the administrative problems. Psychiatric assessments were done under contract instead of as part of an ongoing project. The project's case manager and skills trainer positions at Tender Mercies, Inc., were never filled, staff turnover was high, and the staff who were hired did not perform their jobs according to the proposal, despite ongoing efforts to explain and reiterate the importance of these services both to the research project and to the clients.

Case managers and skills trainers in both the transitional and permanent programs reported infrequent contacts with clients despite their small caseloads. Landlords for the permanent apartment sites complained to the HCCMHB's Housing and Residential Services Program that clients were being left on their own without the promised supports from case managers. Clients were not "graduating" from either of the programs at anticipated rates. The direct service program staff, particularly in the permanent program, did not appear to have discussed or developed criteria or guidelines for determining when clients had achieved functional status that would indicate that they were ready to "graduate", i.e., be transferred to community support services. Those clients who *did* graduate, particularly from the transitional program, reported that they had not been advised of permanent housing options other than those operated by Tender Mercies, Inc.

As these service implementation problems became apparent, HCCMHB personnel took a more direct role in training the agency staff to provide the supportive services as intended under the grant, and in assisting them in establishing guidelines for graduation. Despite these efforts, the direct services provided to clients in both programs could be described as minimal, at best. The apparent lack of any sense of obligation to the clients or the program by the direct service workers was the most troubling aspect of the entire project.

Research Implementation Issues

The two research implementation problems identified by the NIMH site visit team members who recommended project termination were: 1) recruitment of clients to the project programs was well behind the proposed and projected figures; and 2) random assignment of.clients and baseline data collection procedures were determined to be ineffective, unscientific, and inconsistent with the other study sites, although they followed the protocol established in the original project proposal. Although these were identified as research problems, they cannot be totally separated from the administrative and service problems discussed previously.

By the end of the first year of project implementation, it was apparent that the numbers of clients being served by the programs were well under the projected figures – only about half of what had been anticipated. This was primarily due to the administrative and service provision problems previously discussed, but events beyond the program's control also contributed to the delay in filling the study beds. A fire occurred in one of Tender Mercies, Inc.'s residential buildings during the start-up phase of the project. Damage to that building necessitated use of study beds in the transitional program to temporarily house the victims, which delayed the recruitment of study subjects.

The eligibility assessment process itself added to the problem of study beds being filled by ineligible clients. Study participants were recruited mainly from shelters by an outreach worker who made an initial assessment of their homelessness and psychiatric eligibility. The outreach worker was a Tender Mercies, Inc. staff member who was familiar with and trusted by members of the homeless population and by providers of services to the homeless population in the Cincinnati area. After the outreach worker made the initial assessment that a person met eligibility requirements for the study and that person gave, in writing, informed consent to participate in the study, he or she was then randomly assigned by HCCMHB personnel to one of the two study programs. If there was a vacancy in the assigned program, the client was moved into that program. If there was no vacancy, the client was put on a waiting list until a vacancy became available. Once a vacancy was available, the standardized psychiatric (SCID) assessment was completed by the PPSI contract service and if the client was confirmed as being eligible according to psychiatric diagnosis, he/she entered the program and a baseline interview was completed by a project research associate from the HCCMHB.

The intricacies of coordinating the different project agencies and their functions in the process of engaging and assessing the study eligibility of the multi-problem target population members led to problems, particularly in the start-up phase of the project. Homeless persons who *appeared* to be mentally ill and in immediate need of services were sometimes moved into study housing before the psychiatric assessment was completed. Some of these persons were subsequently assessed by the SCID as having substance abuse problems rather than severe mental illness. Clients dislocated by the fire and other clients found to be ineligible for the study were not relocated to other housing as quickly as planned. Tender Mercies staff appeared reluctant to discharge them even when this basically involved transferring them to other agency housing. This slower than anticipated turnover of clients was a major problem to the research component.

The second research problem identified by the NIMH site visit team was that clients were randomly assigned and admitted to the programs before the baseline interview was conducted. Although this protocol followed the project proposal, it was inconsistent with the protocol followed at the other study sites. Researchers at the other sites conducted the baseline interview before clients were admitted to the program. This protocol was not followed at the Cincinnati site, initially because project personnel felt that *immediate* access to housing options was an important aspect of recruiting study participants. The outreach worker could offer potential study participants a place to live at the time of recruitment, not two or three weeks later.

Outreach, diagnostic assessments, and client interviews were conducted by three separate individuals from three different organizations. There was sometimes a two or three week lag between the time a participant was recruited through outreach and moved into housing and the time the SCID psychiatric assessment could be scheduled and completed to confirm eligibility. After that, the baseline interview was conducted for eligible study participants. Scheduling of the SCID assessment was an ongoing problem that was addressed on a number of occasions throughout the life of the project.

The implementation problems which led to defunding of the project after two years permeated the entire project. The administration, service provision, and research implementation problems were intertwined at all levels of the project.

PROJECT RESULTS

Despite the difficulties encountered in implementing the service and research plans, useful service information was gained from the project. First, information was obtained about the characteristics of mentally ill persons who become homeless in an area such as Cincinnati which is relatively rich in community mental health resources and housing options for this population. Compared to the other five study sites, there were many more "permanent" housing options available to study clients.

Characteristics of Study Subjects

Demographics: Fifty-eight eligible persons were admitted to the study; 39 of those persons were followed for a one year period. The clients who completed the one year data collection process were divided fairly evenly between the two programs, with 21 (46%) assigned to permanent housing and 18 (46%) assigned to the transitional program. Seventy two percent of the project clients were male. Forty-six percent were African American (compared to approximately 39% of the city population). Sixty-two percent of the participants reported that they were born in Hamilton County; 41% reported that they had siblings living in the county. The study participants ranged in age at admission from 20 to 65, with a mean age of 34. Most (59%) reported living on disability income: SSI (36%), SSDI (13%), or Social Security benefits (10%); 15% received social welfare benefits.

Diagnoses: The majority of the participants were diagnosed as having schizophrenia or other psychotic disorder (64%); the other 36% were diagnosed with major affective disorders: depression, bipolar disorder, or dysthymia. Over half (51%) were also diagnosed with substance abuse disorders: 31% were found by the SCID to have alcohol abuse or dependence; 20.5% were found to have other drug abuse or dependence.

Homeless status: Forty percent of the study participants were staying in homeless shelters just prior to entering the study programs; 17% came directly from hospitals or mental health crisis care facilities; 16% reported living on the street just prior to entering the program. The others were living with friends or family or in other temporary residences prior to entering the program.

A third of the participants reported having been homeless before the age of 18. Thirty-five percent reported having been homeless for fewer than three months in their lifetime; 26% reported lifetime homelessness of over 3 months but less than 1 year; 39% reported having more than 1 year of time spent homeless.

Fifty-five percent of the participants reported that they had initiated their move from their last place of residence because of dissatisfaction with roommates or other aspects of the residence; 41% reported that they had been asked to leave their last place of residence because of non-payment of rent (7%) or disruptive behavior (34%).

Abuse histories: Over one-third (39%) of the study participants (56% of males; 21% of females) reported being physically abused as children, i.e., having a non-accidental injury resulting in a bruise, burn or abrasion inflicted upon them by an adult parent or guardian. Twenty-six percent of the male participants and 21% of the female participants reported having been sexually abused as children, i.e., forced intercourse by an adult.

Family contacts: Sixty-one percent of the participants reported that they talked to a family member at least once a month or more frequently; 42% got together with a family member at least once a month. Sixteen percent reported no family contact; 26% did not get together with their families.

Feasibility of Supported Apartments for Target Population Members

One of the more positive aspects of the study was the indication that supported community living is a feasible option for members of the target population of homeless persons with severe mental illness. The study participants met the strict eligibility criteria: they were diagnosed with severe psychotic or affective disorders and they were a mix of recent and long-term homeless.

Despite the severity of the participants' problems and the already mentioned problems in service implementation, of the 39 participants followed for the one year period, 27 were living in their own apartments one year after program admission. Five (13%) of the participants were residing in mental health agency supervised housing, 4 (10%) ended up back on the streets or in shelters, 3 (8%) were in psychiatric hospitals, and 1 was in jail. Twelve (31%) were still residents of Tender Mercies, Inc., one year after admission: 9 in the permanent program and 3 in the transitional program.

Identified Service Gaps in the System

The project implementation problems corroborated other indicators of service gaps in the mental health system. A major problem identified by county case managers is the lack of substance abuse treatment options for persons with mental illnesses: current options for substance abuse treatment are not geared to persons with mental illness. As stated previously, eligibility criteria for the study limited participation to persons with *severe* mental illness. Of 32 persons who were found to be ineligible for the study but who were recruited and assessed for participation on the basis of their homeless history and *apparent* mental illness, 20 (62.5%) were diagnosed by the SCID as having primary diagnoses of alcohol or drug related disorders (i.e. abuse or addiction), but *no qualifying psychiatric disorder*. The psychiatric eligibility criteria for Hamilton County's Mental Health Board-funded SA/MI (Substance Abuse and Mental Illness) treatment program for dually diagnosed persons are similar to those of the study – clients must have a major mental illness in addition to their substance abuse diagnosis – so if they were not eligible for the study, they would not be eligible for the SA/MI program either. However, it is likely that the behaviors or characteristics which led the study outreach worker to believe that these persons were exhibiting symptoms of severe mental illness would also lead most substance abuse treatment facilities to reach the same conclusion. Thus, these persons are "not mentally ill enough" for the dual diagnoses programs, but they are "too mentally ill" for most substance abuse treatment programs.

A second gap identified by some of the clients was that their less "major" problems, such as problems with family relations and/or victimization issues, were not being addressed by therapy or counseling. This is an understandable state of affairs given the high level of other needs of these clients and the available resources. However, mental health professionals may have a tendency to categorize clients with severe mental illness as being most able to benefit from medication and case management services and less able to benefit from "cognitive" treatment approaches.

Although the proposed study questions could not be answered and valid comparisons of the study groups could not be made, useful information was obtained from the data collected for the study. However, many of the lessons that may be learned from the project and its demise come from retrospective analysis of the project implementation problems and their causes. Below are some of the recommendations for future administrators of research projects.

RECOMMENDATIONS

Better communication, cooperation, and coordination among the project components were definitely needed for the project to meet its originally proposed objectives. Coordination of the project responsibilities of the various agencies involved was more complicated than it appeared at the time the proposal was first conceived. The effects of the changes in service agency leadership were more problematic than project administrators at the HCCMHB initially recognized. Many of the project start-up problems were beyond human control, but better coordination and administration of the effort certainly was possible.

Recommendations for future research projects involving collaboration among agency programs:

Assign a full-time Research Project Director whose role is to administer the project and monitor its implementation. This person would report to the Principal Investigator. The division of labor and responsibilities among the various project components, i.e., research, psychiatric assessment, service delivery, leasing of permanent housing sites, seemed to be a rational plan given the legal restrictions prohibiting direct service administration by the HCCMHB and its employees as well as the non-project obligations of the Principal Investigator and the other project administrators at the HCCMHB. However, project personnel at all levels could have benefitted from more frequent reminders that the project was primarily a research project with service components rather than a service project with research components. The separation and compartmentalization of research and service activities was not conducive to effective communication of the project's research priorities. A full-time Research Project Director would have been able to give the project implementation and coordination of the various components more focused attention and probably would have identified and addressed the problems more quickly.

Centralize project authority regarding research by having all project service personnel meet directly with the Research Project Director on a regular basis, instead of relying on agency administrators to understand and relay information and protocol to their supervisees.

In retrospect, the project administrators at the HCCMHB probably should have used the contractual agreement to insist that the Executive Director at Tender Mercies, Inc., either a) attend the planning and monitoring meetings on a more consistent basis and provide more detailed and concrete updates on program implementation, or b) allow the project administrators to participate in hiring and training a new program director for the study programs. The HCCMHB project administrators should have insisted on participating in the recruitment and initial orientation of the direct service workers hired specifically for the Project programs at Tender Mercies, Inc. In particular, recruitment of students from social work or psychology programs at local universities to fill these positions was an option that went largely unused. Participation in the hiring process might have allowed for more direct communication of service expectations in the programs, more consistent training of service staff, more centralized coordination of services, and a more global monitoring of the implementation of the services and the research protocol. In this specific case, it also might have helped to foster more identification with the research project and more of a sense of obligation to follow the project service guidelines among the case managers and skills trainers at Tender Mercies. As it was, the Executive Director and initial program director for the two Project programs appeared to resent any "encroachment" on their authority by the HCCMHB, despite the fact that they had a contract to provide specific services and were, in effect, violating that contract. More of a team effort would have been helpful.

Have project research associates conduct all research procedures involving study subjects: recruitment, informed consent, both psychiatric and homelessness eligibility assessments, and client interviews. The outreach worker from Tender Mercies could have done the initial outreach to clients but the final recruitment responsibility could have rested with the research associates. The research associates could have received SCID interview training from PPSI. In retrospect, this division of responsibilities was the main factor to which the project's research implementation problems can be attributed.

CONCLUSIONS

The difficulties experienced by the Cincinnati site researchers were not unique, as many persons who have attempted field research in social service agencies and other "real life settings" will attest. McAuliffe and Ashery (1993) provide a good overview of some of the problems associated with conducting clinical research in outpatient psychosocial treatment facilities for drug abusers. Parallels to the problems they identify, including "conflict between research and clinical needs" (p. 38), difficulties in "administering a large, complex organization over a substantial period of time" (p. 35), and need to make adjustments to treatment and research protocols, can be found in the mental health residential service setting.

Social service direct service providers have traditionally viewed empirical research using their clients as subjects as being more harmful than helpful both to the clients and to the service providers. Agency personnel at the administrative and managerial levels appear to perceive research and program evaluation efforts as useful tools for service planning and quality assurance; direct service workers appear still to perceive research efforts as annoying at best. McAuliffe and Ashery (1993) suggest that having a greater role and participation in the planning and dissemination of research efforts would foster more interest in and commitment to these efforts by direct service providers.

In the course of this chapter, a number of implementation problems have been identified and recommendations made for future researchers. The difficulties in developing, administering, and completing a field research project have been discussed. The caveat "timing is everything" seems particularly appropriate to the Cincinnati project – the project's size and time constraints left a very small margin for error in implementation. The complexities of coordinating an effort which required the commitment and cooperation of staff and administrators from three separate agencies offered many opportunities for error. The major administrative changes experienced by at least two of the agencies increased this potential for encountering difficulties.

It should also be recognized that the recommendations made for future projects will not necessarily be any easier to implement than were the original project plans. Finding an experienced, qualified, and competent full-time Research Project Director willing to commit to a "soft money" position for a one to three year period is a prospect that is easy to recommend but difficult to put into practice. The time constraints associated with the development of proposals and their implementation if funded leave little time to elicit as much participation in the planning phases from direct service workers as would be ideal to foster feelings of "ownership" and commitment to the research aspects of the project. The traditionally high rate of staff turnover at social service agencies adds to this problem, as new workers must be recruited and trained throughout the life of the project.

Despite the difficulties encountered in implementing the Cincinnati Project, the HCCMHB administrators believe that field and service oriented research is crucial to the improvement of mental health services at all levels of administration: state, county, and agency. Our community has received substantial benefits from this project both in terms of funding for additional services for homeless persons with severe mental illness and increased knowledge about the local homeless population and its mental health and other service needs. The establishment of more cooperative working relationships among administrative bodies, service provider agencies, and academic institutions should be encouraged and fostered by grants for research efforts focusing on the common goals of developing and improving models of service provision to various client groups.

REFERENCES

American Psychiatric Association. (1987). Diagnostic and statistical manual of mental disorders-III-R. Washington, D.C.: Author.

Appleby, L., Slagg, M.S. & Desai, P.N. (1982). The urban nomad: a psychiatric problem. Current Psychiatric Therapy 21:253–261.

Bachrach, L.L. (1982). Young adult chronic patients: an analytical review of the literature. Hospital and Community Psychiatry 33:189–197.

Baxter, E. & Hopper, K. (1984). Shelter and housing for the homeless mentally ill. In H.R. Lamb (Ed.), The homeless mentally ill. Washington, D.C.: American Psychiatric Association, 109–140.

Carling, P.J. (1984). The National Institute of Mental Health Community Support Program: Emerging issues. A report of the NIMH/CSP program review. Rockville, MD: National Institute of Mental Health.

Carling, P.J. & Ridgeway, P. (1989). A psychiatric rehabilitation approach to housing. In M.D. Farkas & W.A. Anthony (Eds.), Psychiatric rehabilitation programs: Putting theory into practice (pp. 28–80). Baltimore, MD: The Johns Hopkins University Press.

Goldfinger, S.M. & Chafetz,L. (1984). Residential instability in a psychiatric emergency setting. Psychiatric Quarterly 56:20–34.

Lamb, H.R. (Ed.)(1984). The homeless mentally ill. Washington, D.C.: American Psychiatric Association.

Levine, I.S. (1984). Service programs for the homeless mentally ill. In H.R. Lamb (Ed.), The homeless mentally ill. Washington, D.C.: American Psychiatric Association, 173–200.

McAuliffe, W.E. & Ashery, R.S. (1993). Implementation issues and techniques in randomized trials of outpatient psychosocial treatments for drug abusers. II. Clinical and administrative issues. American Journal of Drug and Alcohol Abuse 19(1):35–50.

Ohio Department of Mental Health. (1988). Housing-as-housing discussion paper. Columbus, OH: Author.

Spitzer, R.L., Williams, J.B. & Gibbon, M. (1986). Instruction manual for the structured clinical interview for DSM-III-R (SCID). 5/1/86 Revision. Biometrics Research Department: New York State Psychiatric Institute.

Stroul, B.A. (1988). Community support systems for persons with long-term mental illness: Questions and answers. Rockville, MD: NIMH Community Support Program.

Turner, J. & Ten-Hoor, W.J. (1978). The NIMH community support program: Pilot approach to a needed social reform. Schizophrenia Bulletin 4:319–349.

9

The Present and Future of Innovative Programs for the Homeless Mentally Ill

JAMES W. THOMPSON and
WILLIAM R. BREAKEY

Having read the papers in this book describing innovative programs for those who are homeless and mentally ill, we are both impressed and sobered.

We are impressed, first, that this field has come a long way in a short time, a good example of a rapid services research response to a perceived need for information about what does and does not work. The McKinney projects were all innovative, but perhaps more important, they were all bold. They attempted to assemble seemingly diverse pieces from CMHCs, consumer advocacy, mobile treatment, housing services, etc., into coherent programs. As we have seen, some were more successful than others in this effort. But even in those which were least successful, there is a wealth of information on how to undertake a study of this sort – and how not to.

But we are also sobered in our response to these stories, for even though much has been accomplished in a relatively short time, there is much more that must be learned about how most effectively to meet the needs of mentally ill homeless people. Even in the most successful McKinney projects, we often do not know for sure what were the keys to that success. And in the projects that had problems, we do not know in every case what were the origins of these problems. We will know much more when the data from the projects are presented in full. However, in terms of understanding basic issues such as the most effective program structure, how to choose patients for particular programs, and what to use as the measures of "success", we are in many ways still at first base.

This final chapter will attempt to synthesize what has been learned in the McKinney projects about developing and evaluating innovative treatment programs for homeless persons with mental illness, and will point towards needed future research. It does not provide a critical review of each chapter, but rather draws upon this body of work to illustrate where the field is at present and where we believe it needs to go. We will refer to each project by its location, distinguishing the two New York Projects as "NYC-State" (David Shern & colleagues) and "NYC-Columbia" (Elie Valencia & colleagues).

The experiences of the six research teams have not only confirmed and advanced our understanding of how homeless people can best be served, they have also confirmed much of what had been learned earlier about homelessness and homeless people. The ubiquity of alcoholism and other substance use disorders, the high prevalence of HIV related disease, the "treatment resistant" nature of some of the individuals served in these programs, and their wide ranging needs are mentioned again and again.

The experiences described here also amply confirm what has been stated before, that while housing is obviously necessary to solve the homelessness crisis, housing alone is not sufficient to meet the needs of severely disabled people such as those served in these model programs. This being said, however, it is noteworthy that the major problems identified in these chapters do not include the pharmacologic management of these chronic and disabling illnesses. Pharmacologic treatments, when properly applied by a psychiatrist and when complied with by the patient, are sufficient to control symptoms in most patients. Rather, the problems identified herein relate to the multitude of other needs presented by patients. These needs, which include counseling, education, rehabilitation, and basic human needs, must be part of an overall treatment approach. With regard to these other needs, the experts on the study research teams have reemphasized many important principles of service provision to homeless people. In addition, they have articulated issues concerning the staffing of programs for homeless individuals, and have clarified many key issues in conducting services research with this population.

THE PHILOSOPHY OF THE PROGRAMS

The first generation of homeless service programs focused on the initial stages of engagement and basic service delivery, with the development of outreach programs and shelter-based clinical services. This next generation of innovations focused on the later stages, i.e., moving homeless people with mental illnesses beyond the immediate treatment situation into housing, and integrating them into the community.

Empowerment

Each of the demonstrations to some extent supported the philosophy of empowerment. One manifestation of this orientation was in the emphasis on client self-determination. NYC-State emphasized client preferences (hence, their program name: "Choices"). In doing so, they maximized continuity and accountability. They found, as has been noted in previous work, that patients more readily accepted services responsive to their self-defined needs and placed more emphasis on meeting basic needs than on addressing mental health concerns.

Baltimore's overall view of empowerment was not so much to emphasize patient preferences (though they did indeed take such preferences into account). Rather, empowerment was operationalized as more of an attitude that clients were competent individuals who were able to meaningfully participate in decisions about their care. San Diego also believed in empowerment, but took a stance which balanced patient leadership and staff control, feeling that there is a need to integrate social control with clinical and social support.

In Boston, empowerment was translated into client control. The Boston program embodied a strong philosophical bent towards a consumer run program. In comparing "evolving consumer house-holds" and independent living, they note that there is a great deal of ambivalence in the field about group homes "run" by consumers, and described the balancing act necessary to achieve a compromise between giving residents total control and respecting the staff's need to act responsibly. We believe this balancing act to be quite important. After all, if disabled adults could simply be handed the keys to the group home, with no input from staff, then housing programs for such patient groups would not be needed. Indeed, the Boston staff found it hard to put this version of empowerment into practice. The idea that the "staff works for the clients" sounded good, but operationalizing this was quite problematic. In part, this was probably because that ideal was not literally true: the residents did not hire the staff, did not pay them, and could not fire them. Also, a paradox existed in that the residents needed to move towards more autonomy, but needed staff help to do so. Any staff help that was given, however, could be construed as lessening autonomy. There was one other area of concern with regard to client control raised by the Boston group. In a separate publication (Schutt & Goldfinger 1996), they indicated that there was a high correlation between substance abuse and the desire of patients for independent living. Since they also found that substance abuse uniformly caused problems for clients in their ability to maintain stable community housing, they question whether for these individuals, empowerment, in terms of independence in living arrangements, is therapeutically positive.

There are several general lessons to be taken from these efforts to empower patients. First, there is a need to be clear about the definition of empowerment: does it mean "handing over the keys" and assuming that the patients will do fine? (In which case, it's difficult to see the need for more than a clerical staff to do the paperwork.) Or does this mean the active participation of patients in treatment planning; involving consumers as staff members; being respectful of patient preferences; treating patients as competent individuals;

or still another definition? Second, how does a particular definition
of empowerment translate into programming? Is this translation
actually therapeutic for the patients? Finally, professionals do not
empower clients by dis-empowering themselves. As one investigator stated, "some of those keys are mine, and I have a responsibility
to keep them". True empowerment empowers everybody involved.

Continuity of Care

NYC-Columbia, along with Boston, emphasized continuity of care,
also a cardinal virtue of PACT and similar programs (Stein & Test,
1980). Insuring continuity of care has long been a major challenge in
health care programs for homeless people. The Baltimore ACT
team, for example, devoted considerable energy to keeping track of
their clients, through inpatient/outpatient continuity efforts and
provision of comprehensive services. Continuity of care was the
specific focus of the NYC-Columbia group, who identified the time
of transition between the shelter and the community as the point at
which patients are particularly at risk of falling between the cracks.
This kind of interface service is not a new idea, but it has seldom
been effectively operationalized.

A major problem in assessing continuity or generalizing from a
particular experience is the difficulty in agreeing on a definition
(Bachrach, 1981). An agreed upon definition is important, as replication of this part of a successful program will depend on being able
to clearly articulate its content. Perhaps these demonstrations help
in the quest for such a definition. What these investigators have
found is that there is a path of services which each patient must
follow in order to succeed. This is defined in part by the providers,
but also by each patient. Indeed, the path may be somewhat different for each person in treatment. It is the job of program developers
to assure not only that certain services are in place, but also to assure (1) that there are linkage and communication mechanisms, and
(2) that there is the flexibility to put the kinds of services and linkages needed by a particular patient into action when and where the
patient needs them. This is a large challenge in times of restriction
and regimentation of health care, but to do otherwise all but insures
that the homeless mentally ill patient will not receive optimal care
and in all likelihood will relapse into homelessness.

Non-Traditional Priorities

Another underlying principle in many of these programs was that
the most important priorities for the clients and therefore for the
service provider may not be those that are traditionally seen as the
top priorities for the mental health service system. For a homeless
person who is mentally ill, obtaining housing is as important as
relief of psychiatric symptoms (Fischer, Colson & Susser, 1996). The
program administrator for funding and political reasons may need

to consider whether a program is primarily a mental health program, serving mental health service goals, or a generic housing program, indistinguishable from other programs serving homeless people, or some combination thereof. Providing housing alone clearly is not enough for a "mental health" program to provide, but where is the line? For example, although the NYC-State program made available a full range of health, mental health, and social services, the program was also designed to meet basic needs for food, respite housing, showers, storage lockers, telephones, laundry facilities. Often, the latter were the priorities of greatest importance to the clients.

So, we enjoin the issue: how much mental health service has actually to be provided to be a "mental health" program? Are "mental health" services even needed for this population? If they are needed, is it better to have separate housing and mental health programs which communicate closely, or it better to have an integrated program which is really both a housing and mental health program? In reading through the various points of view implicit and explicit in the programs described in this book, it appears to us that on this issue the jury is still out.

IMPLEMENTING MODEL PROGRAMS

Infrastructure

Treatment programs do not arise in a vacuum. Unless they are designed to fit well into the context of the entire service system, there will be difficulties in implementation and acceptance. San Diego provides an extensive discussion of the problems they encountered in relating to the overall system of human services in their city, and of the effort which must go into formulating a program that is acceptable to and workable in an existing system. Examples they give are the multitude of definitions of homelessness within the system, and the differing regulations, policies, and philosophies between programs with regard to substance use and criminal behavior.

In the 1980s there was a move in mental health services towards total systems of care. In many communities, however, this did not really happen, and today, all too often, we continue to have a multitude of individual programs which communicate with one another infrequently. Today's funding climate, of "everyone for himself", tends to exacerbate this fragmentation. One thing demonstrated quite clearly by these projects was that for the homeless mentally ill person, a true system can lead to a much better clinical approach, while fragmentation may be disastrous. Instead of calls for new, independent programs, perhaps the next step should be a formal integration of packages of services. Within formal arrangements, disagreements will still arise about definitions and policies, but it should be possible to resolve differences and exert leadership to assist the system to be consistent and coherent.

Relationships with the provider community are also important in working out disagreements. For example, the Baltimore group indicated that referral agencies and the research team often had disagreements on eligibility which had to be resolved. The NYC-State group ran into a more troublesome problem: some referral sources constructed misleading client profiles in order to get the patient accepted for an interview. If there is a poor relationship between the demonstration project and community agencies, such difficulties will be hard to address effectively. The NYC-State team also points to the need for demonstrations to be flexible as they confront resistance in the community. Specifically, they had problems in getting their members into residential programs, a problem that was solved when the demonstration provided post-placement support and guaranteed rent.

Another important lesson is not to draw too sharp a distinction between the "new and improved" demonstration and services that already exist in the community, in order to avoid both destructive competition and the raising of unreasonable expectations as to what the program can achieve. For example the NYC-State group makes the point that early in the project they emphasized differences between their program and existing programs, and oversold the demonstration program. They concluded that it would have been better "to be humbler and more understated". The overall attitude necessary to do research demonstrations in the community was well articulated by the Baltimore group. They state that homeless people and community providers are willing to participate in research if researchers understand and respect the approach to life of homeless people and the nature of the work of community providers.

The Cincinnati project ran into difficulties that occur not uncommonly in systems research, i.e., that changes in the system occur that have nothing to do with the research in hand, but which profoundly affect it. In their case, there were major changes in the administration of the local agencies serving homeless people and in their interest in participating in the research, which contributed in a major way to the abandonment of the project.

STAFFING

Each of the programs had its staffing problems. These problems varied depending in part on whether the program hired professional staff or consumer staff.

Professional Staff

It can be a challenge to entice professionals to work with this difficult population. As an example, Baltimore found it very hard to find a nurse practitioner willing to work in an assertive outreach program with homeless patients. High skill levels are required, and the emotional demands of the job are high, so that working in programs such as these is not unlike working with any chronically ill and disabled population, such as renal dialysis patients. Therefore, various mechanisms such as respite and job rotation need to be worked into the system. Programs for homeless people attract staff whose motivations go beyond the usual ones of money and professional advancement, and who are particularly drawn to caring for the poorest and neediest patients. It takes time to find such people and to build up a team, but once hired they tend to persist and to be very committed to the program and the program's objectives. However, because of the high intensity and this very dedication, there is a significant risk of "burnout" of professional staff and in many cases they will move on to other jobs after only a few years.

The Boston group's unique problem, to put themselves out of a job, has already been referred to. If this model is to be put into effect on a broader basis, the system has to be large enough to assure continued staff employment.

Consumers and Other Non-professional Staff

The NYC-State, Boston, and Baltimore projects employed consumers as staff members. Baltimore also had a family member as a consultant. The NYC-State group notes in a rather understated way that former service recipients who were on the staff sometimes required supervision on boundaries, and that at least early in the program there was a great deal of turnover.

Baltimore perhaps examined this issue in greatest depth in previous work (Dixon *et al.*, 1994). They concluded that consumer-providers have special insights to share and special competencies that professionals lack and thus have an important role in service provision. However, they point out that although these staff persons are not professionals they need some degree of professionalization. This leads to a question: Does this professionalization remove or attenuate some of their special competencies?

Finally, there is another potential problem in mixing the roles of consumers and staff. If differences between roles are minimized, there is the danger of confusing equality as individuals with equality of expertise. For example, consumers clearly have more expertise in understanding the life of a homeless person, but the staff has more expertise in using biopsychosocial interventions to help patients gain greater autonomy. Neither was likely to gain the expertise of the other in full measure. Dixon and her colleagues (1994) expand on this point, as they discuss the role of consumers as part of the service provision team. They address such key issues as the actual day to day roles of consumers in a treatment program; the boundaries between consumer-providers and patients; who should supervise consumer-providers; the impact of the consumer-providers' individual experiences with mental illness on their work; etc. Such questions relate to the discussion of empowerment above, although there are clearly other reasons to hire consumers as staff members.

The areas of consumer involvement and empowerment need some hard thinking to get beyond the "feel good" level of conceptualization. Questions such as those Dixon raise must be tested rigorously, to determine roles for consumers in service programs which can be demonstrated to improve patient outcomes.

It is clear that consumers have a great deal to contribute in the provision of mental health services, just as it is clear that professional training and skills are also essential. The best way of balancing these advantages remains to be demonstrated.

Team Approach

All the projects reported upon in this book demonstrate once again the importance of interdisciplinary teams in treating the severely mentally ill person, particularly those who are homeless, The successes and failures in these programs also point out the difficulties in assembling a team and making it work. In mental health, much lip service is paid to teamwork, but often what is put into place may not at all resemble a team. Several specific lessons are clear. First, a team is something that is built through hard work; it cannot be created out of good intentions or by policy fiat. Second, the patients to some extent must be part of the team, actively involved in planning and executing their treatment. Third, to further the sports analogy, "team" implies that there are several participants who have some basic skills in common, but who also have unique contributions, such as training, talent, experience, or a particular world view. Each team member plays a different position. There can be some overlap in roles, but each team member has specific duties. As previously discussed, the Boston group experienced some difficulties when staff and patient roles became blurred. It is important not to confuse personal worth with expertise and experience.

Building and maintaining an effective team in community mental health has been a challenge ever since the 1960s in the CMHC movement, and remains a challenge today.

Substance Abuse Issues

Substance abuse and dependence were ubiquitous, creating a variety of challenges to the projects. San Diego and NYC-State noted that the staff needed greater skill in treating alcohol and other substance abuse. San Diego tried to provide in-service training to their case managers on substance abuse. Cincinnati also identified dual diagnosis services as a serious gap in their service system.

NYC-State drew attention to the "many questions ... related to the noncontingent provision of resources to individuals with addictions..." (a point also raised by the Boston group). They struggled with the issue of how to provide assistance to individuals that will not be subverted into supporting alcohol or drug habits. This program came to rely on fostering open and frequent communication among staff in managing such patients, and used written contracts between patients and staff. The Baltimore group also confronted the individual choice/enabling dilemma, stating their position as balancing between enabling substance abuse and getting patients into a stable environment where they can work on addiction. NYC-State noted the great deal of staff time that was spent dealing with substance abusing patients, with frequent disagreements between staff, and remarked on how these distractions get in the way of the rehabilitation process.

In summary, the different programs adopted different approaches to dealing with substance abuse, but none of the approaches were ideal. For example, San Diego insisted that their patients be committed to recovery, which greatly restricted their sample size. Baltimore issued no ultimatums and did not require substance abuse treatment. Moreover, they did not address substance abuse immediately with the patient. The NYC-State and Baltimore groups both observe that services needed for homeless substance abusers are different in certain ways from those needed for homeless persons with mental illness. For example there is often direct conflict between the need to get patients into shelters and residential programs and the insistence of many such programs that they do not want substance abusing residents. Most projects found that their patients were not accepted by many shelters, and that other shelters had strict rules on substance abuse.

Clearly, providing services for patients with "dual diagnosis" is one of the major challenges facing our health care system as a whole, and this is reflected in the experiences of the programs reported on here. Much work must be done to design and implement such services. To do this requires individuals who can bridge the gap of ideology and the sense of territoriality between "mental health" and "substance abuse" professionals and groups if these professional arguments are not to get in the way of appropriate care for patients.

THE RESEARCH PROCESS

The Integration of Research and Service Provision

A number of important lessons were learned in these projects about integrating service provision and services research. Each project found that these two agendas were not accepted as equally valid by all those involved. As an example, NYC-State noted that the clinical staff thought that the researchers were intrusive, and the researchers complained about the clinical care in the program, feeling at certain times that the program direction with a particular patient was incorrect. The project directors dealt with this tension in part by increasing interactions between research interviewers and rehabilitation staff, and reconceptualized criticism as valuable program feedback that could be used to change program operations for the better. Baltimore also noted that it is important to keep researchers from becoming part of the intervention, not only to avoid contaminating the research, but also so that a spirit of competition does not arise between researchers and service providers. The San Diego group reported that because of the research protocol, the case managers' caseloads were not under their own control, and interviewers, in order to get the information necessary for the research protocol, had to build relationships with patients, which the case managers viewed as interfering. The project directors took a similar approach to that in NYC-State, in that they stressed daily communication between the service program managers and the research office, and reviewed interviewer activities to maintain the fine line between being researchers and advocates.

Another problem was one that is often troublesome in controlled services research studies – competition between the traditional case managers in the control condition and those in the experimental program (e.g., in San Diego), leading the workers in the control program to modify their practice. The traditional program case managers wanted to do well, and competed with the experimental program to provide good service. Thus the control condition may not necessarily represent "usual treatment", because the staff knows what sorts of things the experimental program is doing and may try to emulate their approach. Such contamination makes it harder to find a positive effect of the experimental program.

The Cincinnati group noted that it is important for researchers to retain control of the process, or the protocol will suffer. In their aborted study, researchers did not have direct control of recruitment, service provision, or transfer to traditional care, since all of these functions were contracted out. Even administration of the SCID was contracted out. The investigators retained responsibility for randomization and data collection, but the lack of overall control contributed to the termination of the research demonstration. On the other hand it can be argued that insofar as control remains with the service providers, the experiment will be more naturalistic, and seemingly less contrived. In addressing this dilemma, it appears that the leadership of the program is very important in setting the tone. If the leadership is clear that the research protocol must be adhered to, but that there will be as little intrusion into the clinical situation as is feasible, things will go more smoothly. If not, there will be continuing problems. The Cincinnati group points out that part time research staff, particularly a part time research director, will have great difficulty in overcoming such problems.

Opinions about research in the larger system are also important. As an example, the Cincinnati group noted that Social Service personnel may see research not simply as a distraction, but as actually harmful to their clients. It is therefore important to work with local agencies to have them understand the value of the research being done, as well as to understand that the demonstration service program would not exist if it were not for the research component.

Methodological issues

Definitions and case identification: Research requires good definitions of cases, interventions, and outcomes. For example, these research groups generally used well delineated definitions for homelessness. However, there are no standard definitions of homelessness. Homelessness is not an either/or condition, and is seldom a steady state (Breakey & Fischer, 1995), so cross sectional definitions are difficult to operationalize. Adding to the difficulty is that some projects, e.g. San Diego and Baltimore, included persons who were "at risk" for homelessness, a very different conceptualization than homelessness per se. In these cases, the intervention could be interpreted as homelessness prevention rather than treatment. Because of these differences in definition, the projects differed somewhat in the criteria they employed for eligibility to enter their programs and comparison between projects is therefore somewhat difficult.

Similarly, rigorous psychiatric case definition is necessary. But here, again, there was wide variation. NYC-State employed a very broad definition of mental illness, and did not use a standard instrument. (They did do a SCID on a subsample). San Diego, on the other hand, had rigorous definitions of mental disorder. Standardization of diagnostic assessment and inclusion criteria across projects would greatly facilitate comparison between programs and generalization to other situations.

Outcome measures: It has been noted that the desired outcomes for programs for homeless people may well be different from those for other populations (Breakey, Susser & Timms, 1994). For example, obtaining a place to live for a homeless person is a key objective which is not likely to be a major objective for judging the success of other mental health programs. This series of projects collaborated on the choice of outcome measures to provide opportunity for comparisons between programs. The measured outcomes, in addition to housing stability, included psychiatric symptom status, physical health status, social functioning, life satisfaction, and measures of substance abuse. The programs reported upon in this book did use a variety of outcomes, and publication of the results of these outcome assessments will be of great interest. Indeed, these research demonstrations may stand as models as to how outcome might be measured in the future.

Randomization: In research of this type random assignment presents major problems. There are many factors, both clinical and political, which interfere with true random assignment. As an example, the difficulties in randomization encountered by the San Diego team weakened an otherwise rigorous design. Some specific problems in randomization noted in the demonstrations were pressure from community agencies to admit particular people to the experimental program; reluctance of some patients to be assigned to one or the other condition; and clinical deterioration of some patients, which led to their termination from the part of the program to which they were randomized. These difficulties became so great in Boston that they decided on a matching strategy as opposed to randomization.

In implementing procedures for random assignment in similar projects, several points must be kept in mind. Staff of other programs in the system and of the demonstration program itself must be educated before the project begins as to the meaning and importance of randomization. In addition, when obtaining informed consent, both conditions must be described to patients as reasonable alternatives for their treatment (being careful not to say that they are equally effective, since the research is precisely to determine whether or not this is true). Finally, procedures should be worked out before the project starts which describe how dropouts from the study will be handled methodologically, so attrition does not seriously compromise the study.

We continue to believe that randomization is a worthy methodologic goal to strive for in research demonstrations. It must be carefully planned, however, if it is to succeed and if the demonstrations are to remain methodologically solid.

Standardization of the intervention: The need to standardize the intervention in some studies came into conflict with the basic philosophy of consumer choice, as discussed above. When patients can choose which services to participate in, one group of consumers may choose services A, B, and C, and another group may choose D, E, and F, so that there is no consistent pattern of intervention. With a sufficiently large sample size some of this variation could be controlled statistically, but large samples are rarely feasible in program demonstrations of this sort. This conflict between consumer choice and the necessities of rigorous research needs to be addressed in future work.

Recruitment and retention: It is a fact of research life that although there are large numbers of homeless individuals, it is difficult to find enough of them in any one area who meet rigorous eligibility criteria to participate in a research project. For example, Baltimore had trouble getting enough patients, and much time and expertise were needed to recruit a sufficient sample. One reason was that many patients were rejected for the study, even though they were very much in need and severely disabled, because the SCID did not identify them as having a severe and chronic Axis I disorder. The San Diego group had a similar recruitment problem.

The experience of these projects seems to call for strategies to increase the number of subjects. Perhaps this could be through multi-site research demonstrations. Although there are major analytical difficulties which must be dealt with in multi-site studies, this would allow for the recruitment of a reasonable number of subjects, provided it is possible to maintain a consistent methodology across sites.

Evaluation and quality assurance: Programs which treat very difficult patients are often highly ideologically driven. That is, much of the staff energy comes from strongly held beliefs about the value of the program. Unfortunately, an all too common attitude in highly ideologically driven programs is "We're too busy performing what we know to be good works to evaluate what we're doing". For similar reasons, some programs may not engage in ongoing quality assurance activities to identify and work out problems. However, research demonstrations are by definition about evaluating the effectiveness of what we are doing. And quality assurance is important because even in a program showing overall effectiveness, there may be many negative (i.e., non-therapeutic) events occurring.

Although there were difficulties in the evaluation of the projects described here, all except Cincinnati did successfully complete their evaluations. Some programs in addition had quality assurance mechanisms in place. In Baltimore, for example, the ACT Team was a clinical program subject to all community mental health regulations. There was regular chart review and the program director and medical director regularly met with staff to review cases. There were also group meetings for treatment planning and "sign out". As noted, such practices are essential to assure quality care, even when the program is in the business of research evaluation.

Ethical Issues

Several ethical issues emerged during the course of these demonstrations. One issue mentioned by several authors concerns control groups. That is, if it becomes clear that the experimental program is more effective in treating this population, is it still ethical to assign people to "usual care" or "traditional case management"? At what point must we offer these effective treatments to everyone? On the other hand, if, for reasons of availability, cost, etc., it is only possible to provide the effective treatment for a limited number of persons, some selection process will have to be implemented, irrespective of research considerations, and random allocation may be as fair as any other selection process.

WHAT REMAINS TO BE DONE?

Although much valuable information has been gleaned from this set of research studies, support is needed for continuing investigation in this area, since many questions remain.

Where to Focus

The NYC-Columbia group makes a convincing argument that we not only need to study programs per se, but also the transition between programs. Especially with this population, which may easily be lost to follow up and may have a difficult time with transitions, such work at the interface between programs is essential.

Another focus clearly needs to be services for persons who are dually diagnosed. Without exception the projects identified this as a glaring lack not only in their programs, but in the service system in

general. Without such services, it will be very difficult to create
optimal programs for such clients.

Longer Term, Longitudinal Studies

The Baltimore group points out that longitudinal studies are needed
if we are to understand the true benefit of novel programs. They are
optimistic that such studies can be done with homeless people,
although these take a great deal of careful planning. They also point
out that most of their patients could not be "stepped down" to less
intensive treatment. (This makes sense, since the reason these individuals were not in traditional care in the first place was their need
for something more intensive.) The fact that these programs will be
long term maintenance programs for some patients makes the need
for longitudinal studies even greater.

Active Factors

Future work must identify the active therapeutic factors in programs which show overall effectiveness. As examples, is more case
management needed, or is a different approach to case management
important? Is the presence of consumers on the staff a key factor? If
so, in what roles? Is patient choice really important in terms of outcome, or is it merely a gesture in response to a current cultural
imperative for empowerment? It would be a great mistake to decide
that a complex program, such as those described, is only effective if
that specific group of services is supplied in that specific way. If the
active and non-active factors can be identified, then possibly the
active factors can be isolated and delivered more cost-effectively
than can the entire package.

Selective Outcomes for Particular Patients

Are there particular patient groups who will benefit from particular
interventions? Perhaps the active factors in a given intervention are
different for different sub-populations. What factors predict good
outcome for particular clients? Studies of this issue will be important for the future, so a more sophisticated approach can be formu-
lated for a given individual. Similar to the active factors discussion
above, being able to target specific interventions for particular
patients would be an optimal use of scarce resources.

Multi-Site Studies

As discussed previously, lack of statistical power is an important
problem with studies of this type. One solution is the use of multi-
site studies which use a common protocol. Such projects are not

easy to design or coordinate, and require very large funding packages, but without them, there may never be enough power to answer some important questions.

Risk Factor Research and Prevention Programs

All of the demonstrations above deal with tertiary prevention (i.e., they aim to prevent relapse). There needs to be attention given, however, to secondary prevention (i.e., early recognition and treatment). As in any prevention program, secondary prevention must be based on knowledge of specific risk factors and on focused interventions which deal specifically with those risk factors. While primary prevention of mental illness is still a far-off hope, it should be quite feasible to develop protocols for testing strategies for the prevention of homelessness in people who are mentally ill. Sufficient risk factor data are available to identify persons at special risk and enable mental health services to provide additional supportive interventions to these patients (Fischer, Colson & Susser, 1996). These are in the future, however, and for now it is important to do as well as we can to fine tune our tertiary services.

CONCLUSION

Successful models are soon lost if they are not disseminated. Every successful research demonstration must devise ways to make others aware of the model and its reasons for success. Many useful innovations have been implemented on a local level, but have now disappeared without a trace.

We hope that this book may help to disseminate the lessons derived from the McKinney projects, may stimulate researchers in this field to go farther with such research, and may stimulate others to become involved in research demonstrations on services to the homeless mentally ill. There is some urgency in the need to further this research agenda. The present national policy direction does not bode well for decreasing the number of mentally ill people who are homeless. We must find out now what works and move ahead to implement programs which are shown to be effective.

REFERENCES

Bachrach, L. (1981). Continuity of care for chronic mental patients: a conceptual analysis. *American Journal of Psychiatry* 138:1449–1456.

Breakey, W.R. & Fischer, P.J. (1995). Mental illness and the continuum of residential stability. *Social Psychiatry and Psychiatric Epidemiology* 30:147–151.

Breakey, W.R., Susser, E. & Timms, P. (1992). Services for the homeless mentally ill. In Thornicroft, G, Brewin, C.R. & Wing, J. (eds.) *Measuring Mental Health Needs*, London: Gaskell.

Dixon, L., Krauss, N. & Lehman, A. (1994). Consumers as service providers: The promise and challenge. *Community Mental Health Journal* 30:615–625.

Fischer, P.J., Colson, P. & Susser, E. (1996). Homelessness and Mental Health Services. In Breakey, W.R. (ed.) *Integrated Mental Health Services: Modern Community Psychiatry*. New York: Oxford University Press.

Schutt, R.K. & Goldfinger, S.M. (1996). Housing preferences and perceptions of health and functioning among homeless mentally ill persons. *Psychiatric Services* 47:381–386.

Stein, L.I. & Test, M.A. (1980). Alternative to mental hospital treatment, I: Conceptual model, treatment program, and clinical evaluation. *Archives of General Psychiatry* 37:392–397.

Index

WA 305
BKE X